Rajvi Shah
Babu GV
Mayur Bhattad

Less Drills, More Smiles

Rajvi Shah
Babu GV
Mayur Bhattad

Less Drills, More Smiles

A Paradigm Shift in Early Childhood Oral Health

LAP LAMBERT Academic Publishing

Imprint
Any brand names and product names mentioned in this book are subject to trademark, brand or patent protection and are trademarks or registered trademarks of their respective holders. The use of brand names, product names, common names, trade names, product descriptions etc. even without a particular marking in this work is in no way to be construed to mean that such names may be regarded as unrestricted in respect of trademark and brand protection legislation and could thus be used by anyone.

Cover image: www.ingimage.com

Publisher:
LAP LAMBERT Academic Publishing
is a trademark of
Dodo Books Indian Ocean Ltd. and OmniScriptum S.R.L publishing group

120 High Road, East Finchley, London, N2 9ED, United Kingdom
Str. Armeneasca 28/1, office 1, Chisinau MD-2012, Republic of Moldova, Europe
Managing Directors: Ieva Konstantinova, Victoria Ursu
info@omniscriptum.com

Printed at: see last page
ISBN: 978-620-8-43675-9

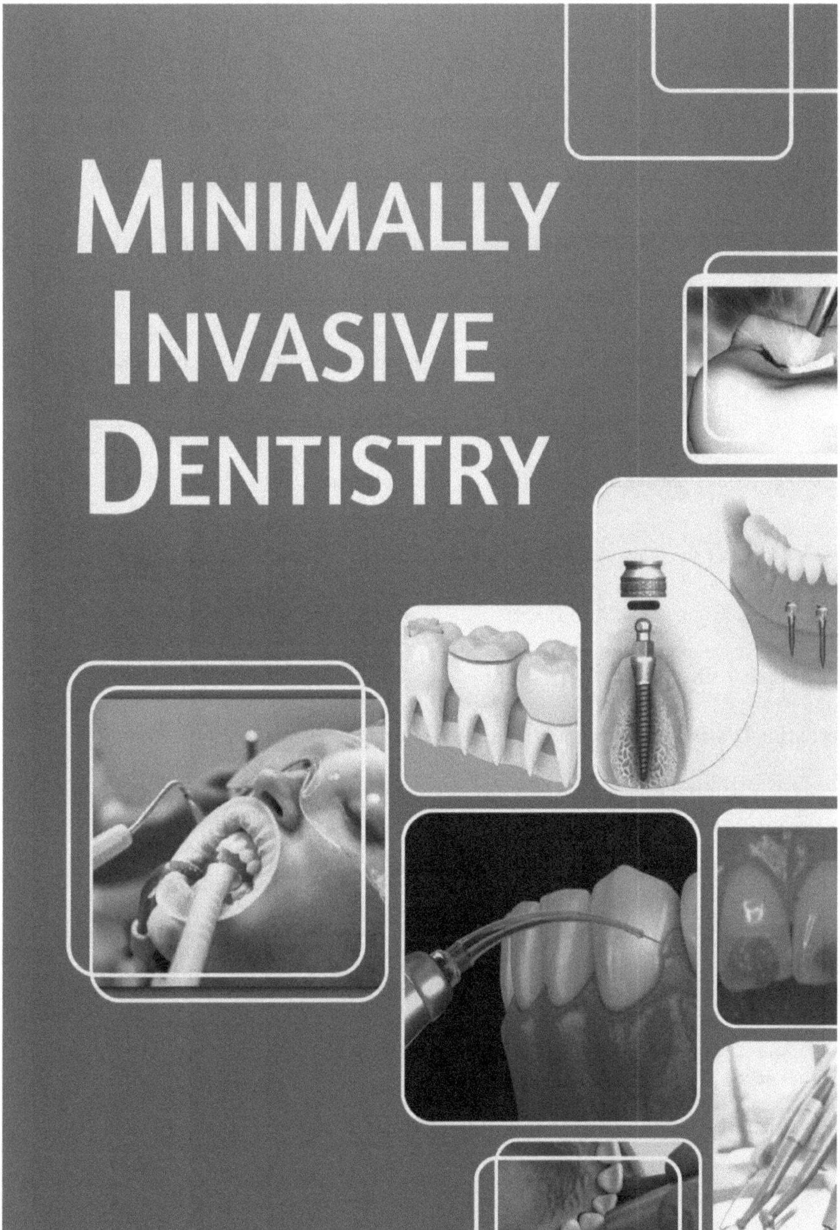
MINIMALLY
INVASIVE
DENTISTRY

Acknowledgement

The starting point to all the achievement is a keen desire to seek knowledge and understanding of the subject. This dissertation is just a small attempt on my behalf to tread the endless path of knowledge. And just like any other journey, this too required timely guidance from many who have been directly or indirectly associated with this dissertation. I would like to take this opportunity to express my heartfelt gratitude to everyone who has supported and guided me throughout my three-year journey in Paediatric & Preventive Dentistry. This academic pursuit has been both enriching and challenging, and I am deeply thankful to all those who made it possible.

First and foremost, I am profoundly grateful to God, the Almighty, for granting me the strength, good health, inspiration, and perseverance. I would like to thank my esteemed guide **Dr. Babu G.V**, Professor and H.O.D, Department of Paediatric & Preventive Dentistry, for his kindness, courtesy, valuable suggestions and inspiration. He has nurtured it with the essentials, leaving no scope for any deficiency.

I owe special thanks to **Dr. Mayur Bhattad,** Professor, Department of Paediatric & Preventive Dentistry, for his unwavering support and encouraging words that have always boosted my work. I am deeply grateful for his support and understanding over these past three years.

I am also thankful to **Dr. Sumit Rajewar** and **Dr. Ankita Chandak,** Senior Lecturers, Department of Paediatric & Preventive Dentistry, for their inspiring guidance and friendly advice throughout the journey.

I would like to thank ***Dr. Vivek Choukse,*** *Dean, Dr. HSRSM Dental College & Hospital, for helping me out with whatever way possible.*

I am deeply grateful to my Grandmother ***Smt. Chandramani Shah****, my Father* ***Mr. Rashmikant Shah****, my late Mother* ***Harsha Shah****, my Uncle* ***Mr. Anish Shah****, and my Aunt* ***Mrs. Jigisha Shah.*** *Thank you for instilling in me the values of hard work and perseverance. Your love, support, sacrifices and unwavering belief in me has been the foundation of all my achievements.*

I extend my heartfelt appreciation to my siblings, ***Ar. Priyal Shah, Er. Jeet Shah,*** *and* ***Ms. Jeenal Shah****, for being my pillars of strength and constant companions throughout this journey. Your unwavering support and shared laughter made this journey easier and more joyful and gave me the confidence to pursue my dreams. Your belief in me is my strength.*

To my friends, ***Dr. Rhujuta Chaudhari, Dr. Pranauti Sonaje, Dr. Bhoomika Kulkarni, Dr. Avinash Sherkar, Dr. Shubham Khandale, Dr. Daksha Soni*** *and* ***CA Pratiksha Soni,*** *your companionship has been nothing short of extraordinary. Your constant encouragement and infectious laughter made this journey truly memorable. From the early days of card playing sessions to the triumphant moments of achievement, your friendship has been a source of inspiration and strength. Thank you for standing by me through it all.*

To my colleagues, ***Dr. Komal Chaudhari and Dr. Keyuri Patil****, I extend my heartfelt appreciation for your inspiring presence and support. I am grateful to my juniors* ***Dr. Samruddhi Bengal, Dr. Apurva Rane*** *and* ***Dr. Shivani Kolhe*** *for their help.*

This dissertation is a testament to the collective effort and support of many individuals. I am deeply indebted to all who contributed to this journey, and I hope to carry forward the knowledge and values you have imparted to me.

Thank you all.

Dr. Rajvi Rashmikant Shah

CONTENTS

INTRODUCTION

Initially, 'Minimally Invasive Dentistry' (MID) was coined to describe the utilization of smaller and less intrusive techniques for addressing dental caries. Presently, it encompasses a more comprehensive philosophy of care that includes assessing individual patient's risk factors, early detection of oral disease, implementation of targeted prevention strategies, and performance of limited surgical procedures tailored to the extent of the disease. Essentially, MID represents a modern medical approach to the treatment of dental caries that emphasizes risk assessment and prioritizing early prevention and intervention over tooth restoration.

MID extends its principles beyond dental caries management and is applicable to various aspects of oral health, including periodontology, oral rehabilitation, and oral surgery. This versatility highlights MID's potential to revolutionize many facets of modern dentistry. One of the pivotal developments contributing to the MID philosophy is the understanding of fluoride's role in retarding carious lesion progression rather than preventing initial development. This knowledge has revolutionized the way dental professionals approach caries management and highlights the significance of post-eruptive fluoride exposure in maintaining oral health.

Dental caries is recognized as a complex disease driven by an imbalance in the mineralization of teeth and the presence of biofilm. Specific bacteria play a role in its development, and lesions form where biofilms are allowed to persist. Effective plaque removal through daily brushing, in combination with fluoride toothpaste, has become a cornerstone in managing carious lesion development worldwide. Advancements in adhesive materials have been instrumental in achieving the main objective of MID, which is to minimize the removal of healthy tooth tissue during treatment. This has led to smaller and less destructive cavity preparations, resulting in smaller restorations.

Dawson and Makinson further elaborated on this approach and introduced the term 'Minimal Intervention Dentistry' in the literature. The International Association for Dental Research (IADR) also organized a symposium in 1995 dedicated to minimal intervention techniques for dental caries, with a focus on Atraumatic Restorative Treatment (ART).[1]

HISTORY & EVOLUTION

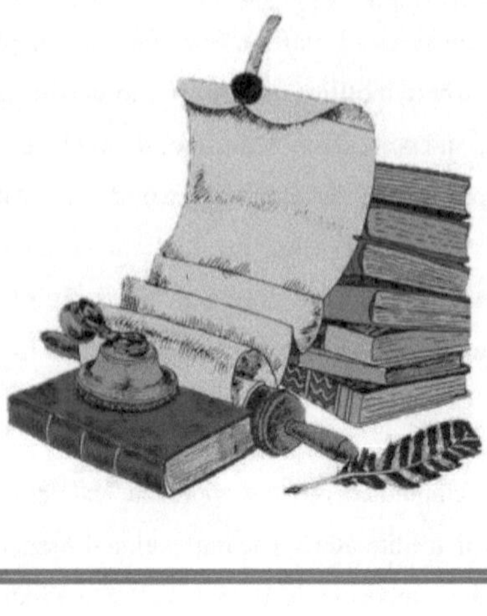

G.V. Black pioneered the concept of minimal intervention in the treatment of dental caries, a departure from the prevailing surgical model of his era, which often relied on tooth extraction or traditional restoration to address clinical symptoms. At that time, dental restorations utilized an alloy prone to rapid corrosion and expansion issues. However, pivotal events unfolded that paved the way for the advancement of dental amalgams and the introduction of bonded restorations. In 1955, Buonocore introduced a technique for etching enamel surfaces to enhance their retention for restorations, while Bowen's invention of adhesive materials in 1962 laid the foundation for minimally invasive preparation techniques.[2]

	Old Model	**New Model**
Dental Caries	Drilling & Filling	Risk Assessment
	Mechanical Retention	Preventive Care
	Extraction	Adhesive Dentistry

" History teaches us that innovation in dentistry, through minimally invasive techniques, not only enhances patient outcomes but also transforms dental practice into a realm of gentle precision and lasting smiles."

Timeline[3] –

- **1890**: Greene Vardiman Black (G.V. Black) introduced principles of cavity preparation that included removing diseased tissue aggressively to prevent recurrence, which was later contrasted by the concept of minimally invasive approaches.
- **1923** : Hyatt Introduced Prophylactic Odontotomy.
- **1928** : Prime Designed a class II cavity that included a narrow, shallow occlusal step and narrow gingival walls inclined to the axial for retention.
- **1932** : Dr. Edwin Fisch, first applied ozone in dentistry.
- **1936** : McGhee in his "Textbook of operative dentistry" advocated a class II cavity in which the buccal and lingual margins converged towards the occlusal .
- **1945** : Air abrasion excavation was originally developed by Robert Black.
- **1955** : Buonocore developed Acid-etch technique for adhesion of resins.
- **1960** : A new understanding of carious dentin emerged where it was identified as two separate carious dentin layers, an outer infected dentin and an inner affected dentin by fusayama using fuschin dye.
- **1962 :** Bowen developed Bonding agent.
- **1963** : Jinks Introduced tunnel preparation.
- **1965** : Owen Developed Bis-Gma resin.
- **1966** : Markley discovered modification of GV black's cavity design.
- **1972** : Wilson and Kent developed Glass Ionomer Cement.
- **1975** : Goldman and kronman Made first attempt to use chemo mechanical removal of caries.
- **1978** : Preventive Resin Restoration was developed by Simonsen & Strallard.

- **1980** : Hunt & Knight developed Tunnel restoration.
- **2007** : CAMBRA was developed by Featherstone.
- **1984**: Introduction of Glass Ionomer Cement by Alan D. Wilson and Brian E. Kent, allowing for atraumatic restorative treatments (ART) in pediatric dentistry.
- **1985**: Concept of Pit & Fissure sealants gained momentum with the aim of preventing caries non-invasively.
- **1992** : Dawson & Makinson gave term Minimally Invasive Dentistry.
- **1994**: The Atraumatic Restorative Treatment (ART) technique, spearheaded by Jo E. Frencken, was introduced, focusing on the removal of decayed tissue using hand instruments and restoring with GIC.
- **1995** : Development of MID approaches : ART was done in 1ST IADR symposium.
- **1997** : Graham mount Proposed a new cavity classification to take into account the changes in caries activity. Carious lesion occurs in 3 sites on the crown or root of the tooth with severity of lesion in 5 sizes (size-0 to size-4).
- **1997** : Bjorndal et al, treated deep/extensive dentinal carious lesions with selective or stepwise which seems advantageous compared with complete caries removal and found selective removable more efficient.
- **1998** : Tooth separation method was given by Hintze et al.
- **1999** : Nyvad Classification was developed.
- **2000:** Sono abrasion was developed by Banerjee et al.
- **2000** : Martin et al applied the term 'Minimal Intervention', 'Minimally Invasive' or 'Preservation dentistry which was earlier named as "Prophylactic Odontomy
- **2001** : The International Caries Detection and Assessment System (ICDAS) was developed.

- **2001**: Development of silver diamine fluoride (SDF) in Japan by Nishino & Yamaga for caries arrest in children, gaining attention globally for its non-invasive properties.
- **2002**: The International Caries Detection and Assessment System (ICDAS) was modified promoting early detection and non-invasive management of caries.
- **2002** : CAMBRA was developed by Featherstone in NUS (National University of Singapore).
- **2003** : Papacarie was introduced by Sao Paulo in Brazil.
- **2003** : Smart burs were developed by SS White dental.
- **2005** : Smiles for life: The AAP and National Interprofessional Initiative on Oral Health (NIIOH) have collaborated to create a formal Oral Health Risk Assessment Tool
- **2005**: Definition of MID was given by Tyas MJ et al.
- **2005** : Cariogram was developed by Douglas Bratthal and associates at the Dental School in Malmo.
- **2006** : Introduction of the Hall Technique by Norna Hall, which involved sealing caries under preformed metal crowns without caries removal.
- **2006 :** Traffic Light Matrix (TLM) developed by the American Academy of Paediatric Dentistry (AAPD).
- **2010**: Laser-based cavity preparation techniques began gaining popularity, allowing non-invasive removal of caries in pediatric patients.
- **2010** : Photothermal radiometry and modulated luminescence was developed.
- **2010 :** Carie care gel was introduced.
- **2011** : The Caries Assessment Spectrum and Treatment (CAST) instrument was first described.

- **2013** : My Smile Buddy is designed for use on a portable interactive multimedia device (Apple i-Pad) that assists the community health worker (CHW) or other peer educators.
- **2013** : Principles of MID were given by Murdoch.
- **2013** : Core principles of MID were given by Walsh.
- **2014**: Introduction of resin infiltration (Icon System by DMG) for managing incipient caries non-invasively.
- **2014** : U.S. Food and Drug Administration (FDA) gave clearance to the first SDF preparation for dental use.
- **2015** : Silver Diamine Fluoride was available for use.
- **2016** : Caries risk assessment for treatment (CRAFT) developed by Dr. Ashwin Javdekar.
- **2016** : BRIX 3000 gel was introduced.
- **2018**: OXIS classification was given by Kirthiga M et al.
- **2018**: Resin infiltration technique was given by Mirsiaghi et al.
- **2020**: Incorporation of Artificial Intelligence (AI) for early caries detection and non-invasive management in pediatric dentistry.
- **2022**: Expansion of SDF globally, with significant research advocating its role as a primary MID tool in pediatric care.
- **2023**: Introduction of bioactive materials like calcium silicate-based sealants for minimally invasive restorative techniques.

CARIES DIAGNOSIS

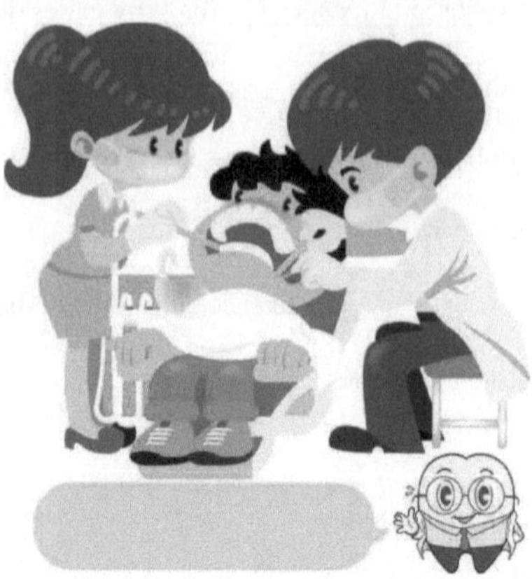

Early diagnosis of dental caries is essential for minimally invasive procedures in restorative dentistry. Dental caries, a microbial disease affecting the teeth's calcified tissues, involves demineralization of the inorganic portion and organic substance destruction. It is now understood as a dynamic process with potential for progression, stabilization, or regression.

The decline in caries prevalence also brings about notable changes in lesion morphology, such as slowly progressive dentinal lesions hidden under apparently intact enamel, often termed **"Coke bottle"** shaped fissure caries.

An effective diagnostic approach for dental caries should enable detection at its earliest stages and allow for the identification of all pathological changes from early demineralization to cavitation. While no single method exists to detect caries on all tooth surfaces, certain technologies show promise in providing higher specificity and sensitivity for early caries detection and quantification. These advancements can aid in the development of more effective preventive or minimally invasive interventions.[30]

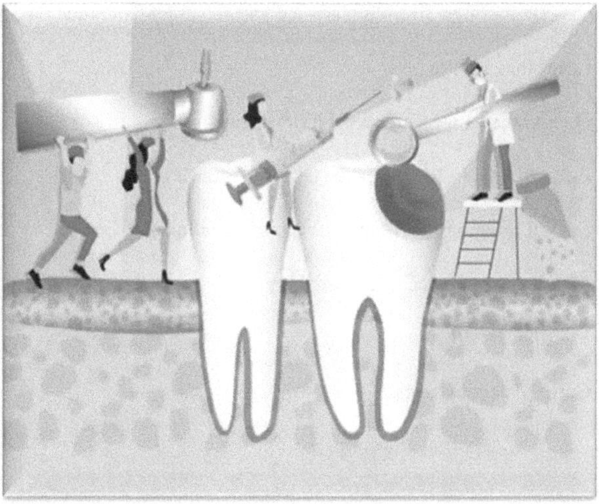

Diagnostic Methods

A. Visual as well as visual tactile inspection.
B. Meticulous clinical visual method.
C. Visual method with temporary elective tooth separation.
D. Visual method with temporary elective tooth separation and impression of the approximal lesion.
E. The radiographic method.
F. Direct magnification technique(DIMA).
G. The digital radiographic method.
H. Digital subtraction radiography(DSR).
I. Optical coherence tomography (OCT).
J. Tuned aperture computed tomography(TACT).
K. Electrical conductance.
L. Electrical impedance tomography(EIT).
M. The alternating current impedance spectroscopy technique (ACIST).
N. Laser fluorescence.
O. Quantitative Light-Induced Fluorescence (QLF).
P. Infrared Laser Fluorescence (DIAGNOdent®).
Q. Digital Imaging Fiber Optic Transillumination(DIFOTI).
R. Magnetic resonance micro-imagery.
S. Microbial testing.
T. Caries detecting dyes.

3.1 Visual as well as visual tactile inspection

Greenverdiman Black, the father of conservative Dentistry in 1924, suggested the use of a sharp explorer. If a slight pull was required to remove the explorer from the tooth surface i.e. if there was a "catch" then the surface was counted as being decayed. Simon in 1956, Gillmore in 1982, Marzouk in 1985 and Sturdevant in 1985 also supported the use of an explorer for caries detection.[30]

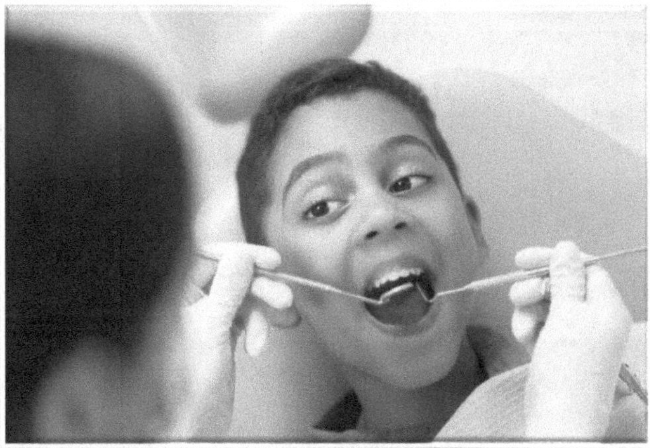

Disadvantage :

The utilization of a probe carries the risk of spreading decay-causing bacteria to different areas. Therefore, there is a growing dependence on visual diagnosis in current practice.

3.2 Meticulous clinical visual method

A thorough clinical examination, conducted meticulously after cleaning, including flossing all surfaces and ensuring thorough drying, will reveal more lesions compared to quick clinical assessments.[30]

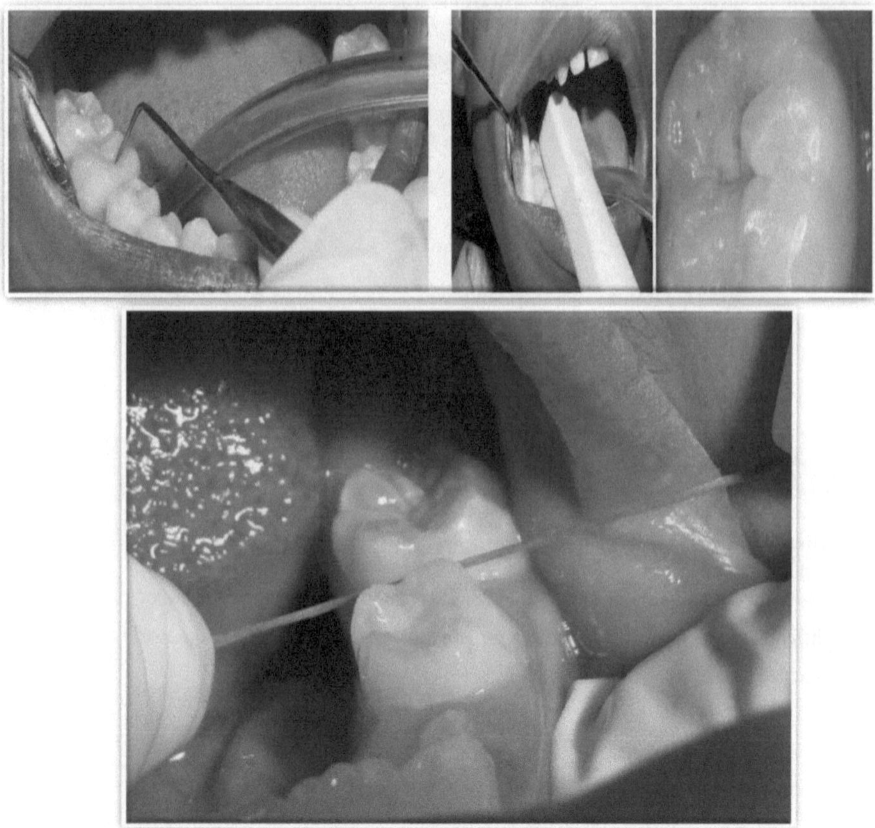

3.3 Visual method with temporary elective tooth separation

Since the last century, the practice of employing bands to create space between teeth for better visualization of the posterior approximal surfaces has been established. This method achieves gradual separation.[30]

Visual method with temporary elective tooth separation and impression of the approximal lesion:

Temporary elective tooth separation, coupled with a localized impression of the expanded interproximal space, enhances the sensitivity of cavitation diagnosis compared to a purely visual separation method. Additionally, this approach offers the benefit of creating a replica for visual monitoring of size changes or even for measuring serial impressions.

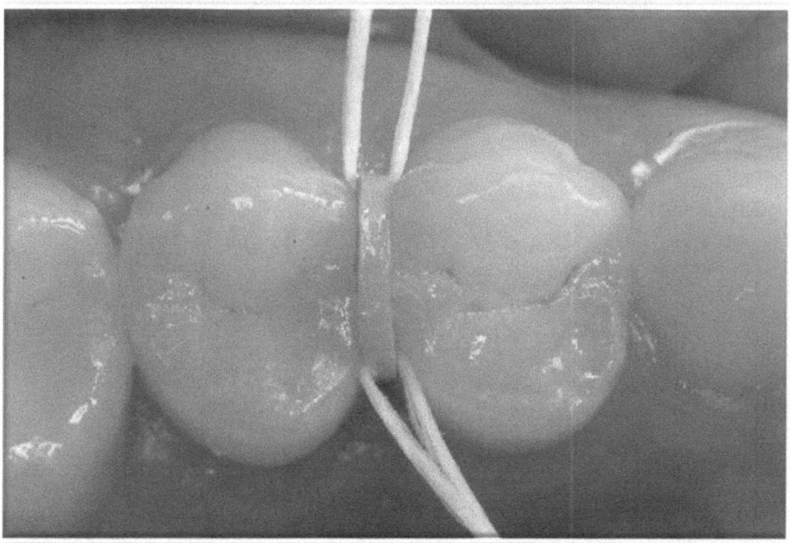

3.4 Conventional bitewing radiographic method

Previously, bitewing radiographs were utilized to identify proximal decay, as caries often develop just beneath the contact point, whether mesially or distally. Presently, these radiographs are also employed to uncover hidden occlusal dentin lesions. However, it's crucial to interpret radiographs cautiously, as they present a two-dimensional representation of a three-dimensional object. Furthermore, it's essential to consider that a substantial mineral loss, typically exceeding 20-30%, is necessary for radiographic detection.[30]

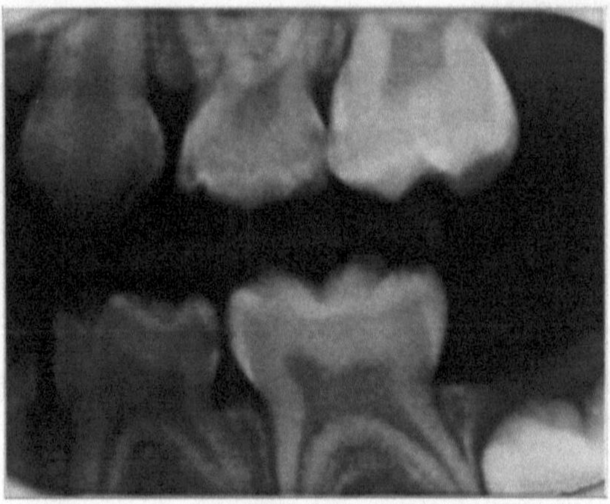

Limitations:

a) Exposure of child to ionizing radiation.

b) Limitations of dental film.

c) Physical limitation based on anatomic consideration.

d) High degree of inter-examiner variability.

e) Amount of labour, time required for processing.

f) Variability in the image produced.

3.5 Direct magnification technique (DIMA)

In dental radiology, the intraoral technique utilizing direct film offers the highest definition in imaging. Conventional dental X-ray tubes typically feature a relatively large focal spot, approximately 700m in diameter. This size can create a "penumbra" effect, leading to decreased contrast, diminished definition, and the occurrence of artifacts. To mitigate this effect, a large focus-to-object distance and a small film-to-object distance are employed.[30]

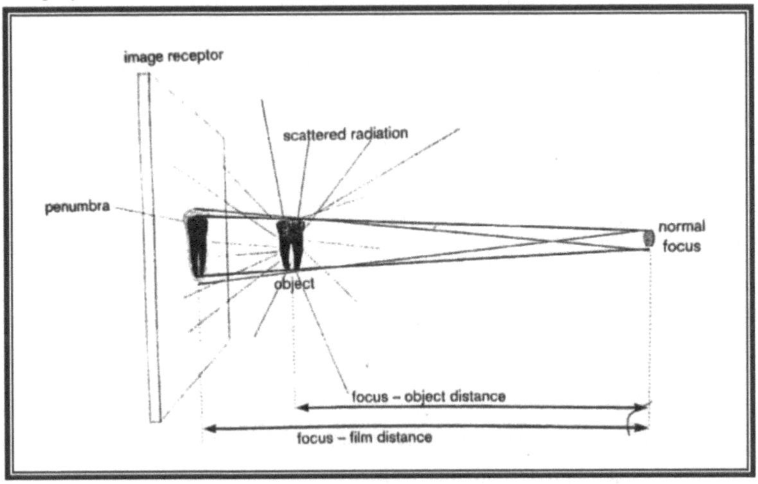

However, this approach can reduce image quality due to scattered radiation from the object. In response to these limitations, the Direct Magnification Technique (DIMA) has been introduced. An essential requirement for implementing the DIMA technique is the availability of an X-ray source with the smallest possible focal spot to generate images without any penumbra.

Principle :-

The DIMA technique employs a fundamentally distinct setup compared to traditional methods. In DIMA, the focus-to-object distance is minimized, while the object-to-film distance is increased. In clinical practice, this method necessitates positioning the focal spot near the object using an intraoral rod anode tube. To achieve high-quality DIMA images, a focal spot diameter of less than 100 is indispensable.

3.6 Digital Radiograph

Digital, filmless techniques for intraoral radiography have been developed for several important reasons[30] :

A. Traditional film absorbs only a small fraction of the x-rays it encounters, resulting in minimal radiation exposure for the patient.

B. Inadequate darkroom practices can result in both excessive radiation exposure and the loss of crucial diagnostic data.

C. Film development is a time-intensive process, and the chemicals used in developer and fixer solutions pose environmental hazards.

Digital radiography is rapidly becoming one of the most sought-after advancements in dentistry, driven largely by enhanced accessibility, performance, and reduced computer costs. Surveys indicate that a significant portion of dentists prioritize digital radiography, considering it a top priority.

Practitioners who have embraced this technology recognize that the quality of images produced is comparable to traditional film. Moreover, they appreciate the advantages it offers, such as improved patient communication and comprehension, time efficiency, reduced radiation exposure, enhanced diagnostic capabilities, elimination or reduction of chemical usage, and more effective marketing for their practice.

Prominent manufacturers of direct digital radiography systems include:

a) Schick CDR, Trex.
b) Trophy RVG, New Image Ni-Dx, Siemens.
c) Sirona Sidexis, Dexis Digital X-ray.
d) Cygnus Ray 2.
e) Sens-A-Ray.

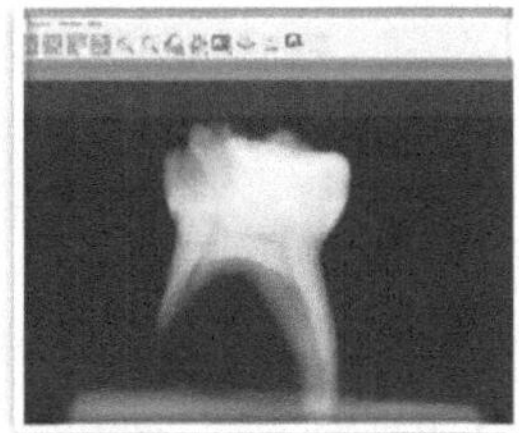

3.7 Digital subtraction radiography (DSR)

A promising approach for identifying diagnostically relevant changes involves subtracting successive standardized radiographs, potentially enhancing the detection of lesions previously challenging to visualize. This technique underpins subtraction radiography. Subtraction images can be generated using photographic, electronic, and digital methods, with Digital Subtraction Radiography (DSR) being widely utilized and popularized within the dental community.

Discrepancies between the images manifest as either darker or brighter regions, depending on the nature of tissue alterations.

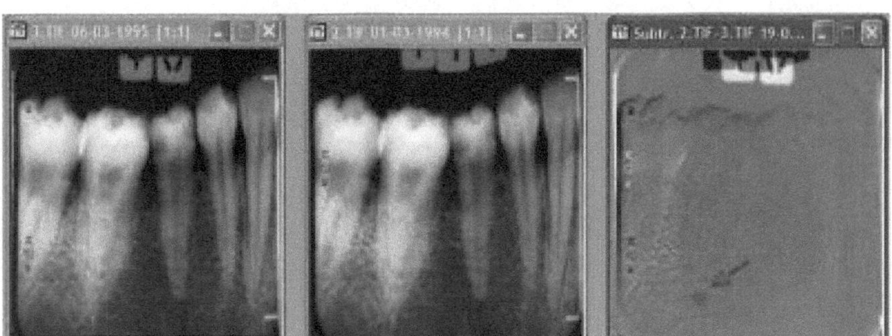

3.8 Optical coherence tomography (OCT)

In traditional plain film radiography, both the radiographic film and the source remain stationary. This setup captures all anatomical structures between the source and the film, often obscuring important diagnostic details. The concept of 'Tomography' initially referred to sectional radiographic methods.[30]

In tomography, the radiographic tube moves synchronously with the film plate but in the opposite direction during exposure. This motion ensures that the image of the selected anatomical plane remains static on the moving film, while shadows from other planes are either blurred or eliminated. Consequently, a tomographic image depicts a specific layer or slice of the structure being imaged.

Optical Coherence Tomography (OCT) is an innovative optical technique for non-invasively imaging biological tissue. It produces high-resolution (less than 20) cross-sectional images of tissue without the need for biopsy. OCT utilizes near-infrared light to capture images, eliminating the risks associated with ionizing radiation present in X-ray imaging.

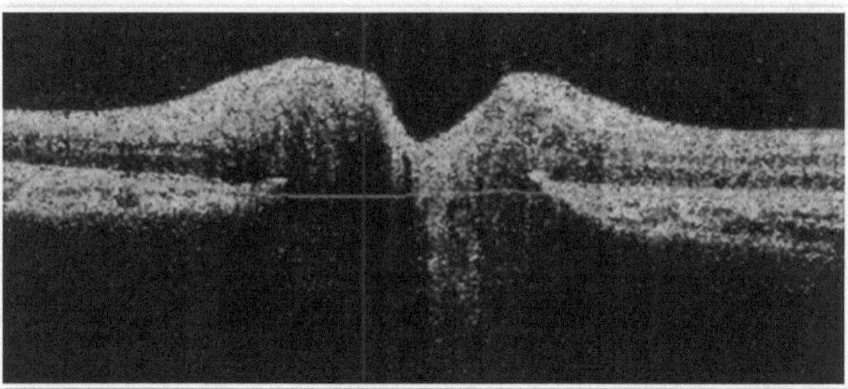

Principle :

Near-infrared light has the capability to penetrate tissue deeply, making it valuable for imaging internal structures. However, a significant portion of this light becomes highly scattered upon entering the tissue, resulting in blurred images in most applications.

OCT employs a white light Michelson interferometer as a gate, allowing it to exclusively detect unscattered "ballistic" photons. This selective detection enables OCT to produce high-resolution images. By discerning between scattered and transmitted or reflected photons, OCT unveils microstructural tissue details.

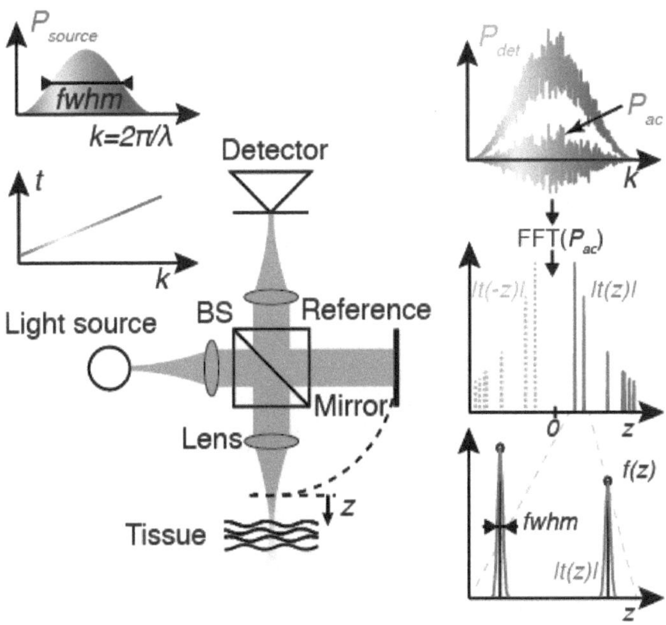

3.9 Tuned aperture computed tomography (TACT)

TACT, which applies the principles of Tomosynthesis in a broader context, shows potential in enhancing accuracy in caries diagnosis due to its 3-D or pseudo 3-D capabilities. To comprehend the principle behind TACT, it's essential to have a brief understanding of related terms such as Conventional Tomography, Computed Tomography (CT), and Tomosynthesis.[30]

Conventional Tomography :-

The development of plain tomography by Zeis des Plantes, further refined by Grossman, resulted in a clinically practical technique where structures above and below the diagnostic focus are deliberately blurred. Rosenberg initially described this method for achieving depth-specific imaging in the maxillofacial region.

One notable drawback of this approach is the apparent blurring caused by the superimposition of out-of-focus structures. Additionally, obtaining multiple slices is often required to ensure thorough sampling of the region of diagnostic interest. Once the patient has departed from the imaging facility, no additional image layers can be acquired, presenting a limitation.

Computed Tomography (CT):-

CT has developed into a remarkably efficient diagnostic imaging method, capable of fully sampling an object by rotating an X-ray source and digital detector around it. By doing so, CT effectively eliminates the superimposition of images from structures above or below the area of interest in the patient, while also offering up to ten times greater contrast resolution compared to conventional tomography.

However, despite these advancements, CT has encountered restricted use in diagnosing numerous common dento-alveolar diseases. This limitation stems partly from the expense associated with CT scanning and also from its relatively limited spatial resolution.

Tomosynthesis :-

The foundational principles of tomosynthesis were initially delineated by Ernst Pohl of Kiel in 1931. Similar to CT, in tomosynthesis, the X-ray source remains fixed in a plane while its position within that plane moves to predetermined discrete sites, typically arranged in a circular distribution. However, unlike CT, the plane in tomosynthesis does not necessarily align with the reconstruction plane.

Its primary advantage over CT lies in its ability to generate an infinite number of laminograms from a finite set of radiographs. This method allows for the retrospective creation of numerous tomographic slices from a limited number of conventional transmission radiographs, provided that the projections are generated from different angles. Additionally, tomosynthesis effectively eliminates noise from out-of-focus structures.

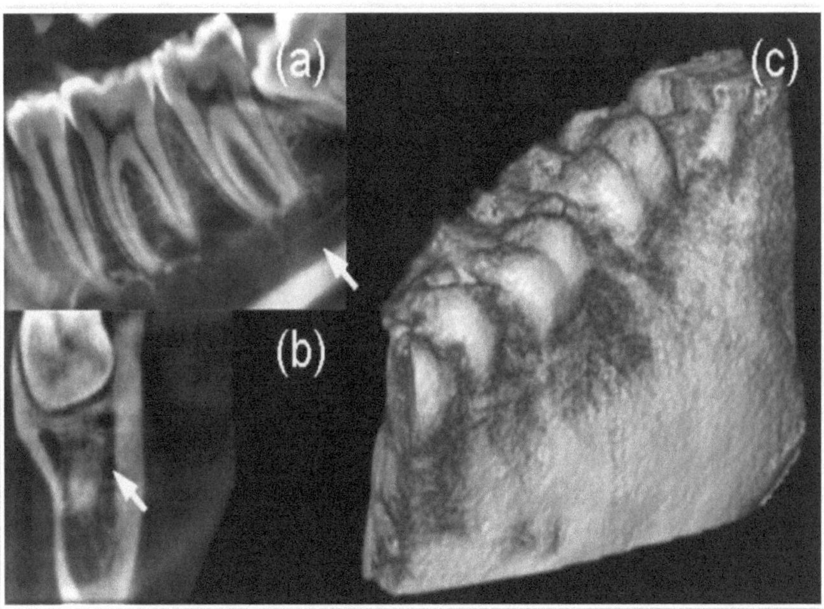

3.10 Electrical conductance measurement

Magitot introduced the concept of using an electrical method for detecting caries in 1987. The underlying theory of Electrical Conductance Measurement (ECM) is based on the premise that healthy tooth surfaces exhibit minimal or negligible conductivity, whereas carious or demineralized enamel demonstrates measurable conductivity, which increases with greater demineralization.[30]

As demineralization progresses, the electrical conductivity of a tooth undergoes changes. A conducting medium covers the entire occlusal surface, and conductivity from this surface to a ground electrode is gauged using a probe. The rise in conductivity is attributed to the formation of microscopic demineralized cavities within the enamel, which become filled with saliva.

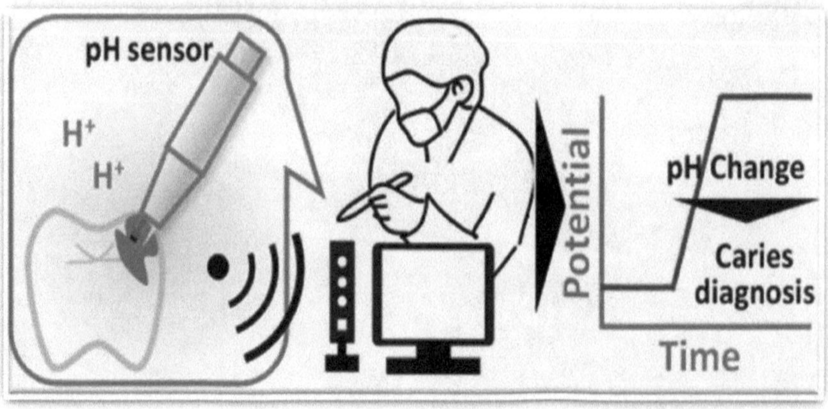

Recently, there has been a renewed interest in electronic resistance measurements, leading to the introduction of two new devices: the Electronic Caries Meter (ECM) from LODE, Gronigen, Netherlands, and the CariesMeter L from Onuki Dental, Japan. These instruments operate on the principle that healthy enamel exhibits high resistance to electric current flow, while porous carious enamel, with its micro-porosities filled with conducting media such as water and saliva ions, demonstrates progressively lower resistance and higher conductance as the lesion advances and expands.[31,32] The meters can be calibrated to assess the depth and extent of caries. However, caution is advised when examining immature teeth (i.e., those with less than 18 months of oral exposure), as readings may erroneously suggest caries when the teeth are actually sound.[33]

One drawback of this system is the need for teeth to be dry, but not desiccated, to prevent current leakage.[34] Optimal results are achieved with a moderated airflow over the tooth surface. While these systems excel in detecting caries in pits and fissures and are relatively accurate in diagnosis, some studies have reported false positive values of up to 23%.[35] Teeth with enamel cracks may yield abnormal readings, indicating caries presence even when absent; however, this feature may prove useful in investigating cracked tooth syndrome, where the crack serves as a conductance pathway containing saliva and oral debris.[36]

Additionally, the ECM may have the capability to detect fissure sealant failures. Variation in results may occur depending on whether alternating current (a.c.) or direct current (d.c.) is used, the selection of fixed or wide-range frequency, and the size of the tip in contact with the tooth.[37] Laboratory experiments employing a.c. current over a wide frequency range have shown excellent results (100% sensitivity and specificity) particularly when assessing electrode conductance over the entire tooth surface rather than at a specific site.[38] Previous experiments have shown a reasonable correlation between readings and histological validation for dentine lesions; however, applying the electrode across the entire surface has proven less effective in detecting early enamel lesions.[39]

Disadvantages:

Abnormal readings may occur in teeth with enamel cracks; however, this characteristic could be advantageous in exploring cracked tooth syndrome, as the crack can function as a conductance pathway due to its presence of saliva and oral debris.[40]

Caution is advised when evaluating newly erupted teeth, as readings may erroneously suggest the presence of caries when, in reality, the teeth are healthy.[41]

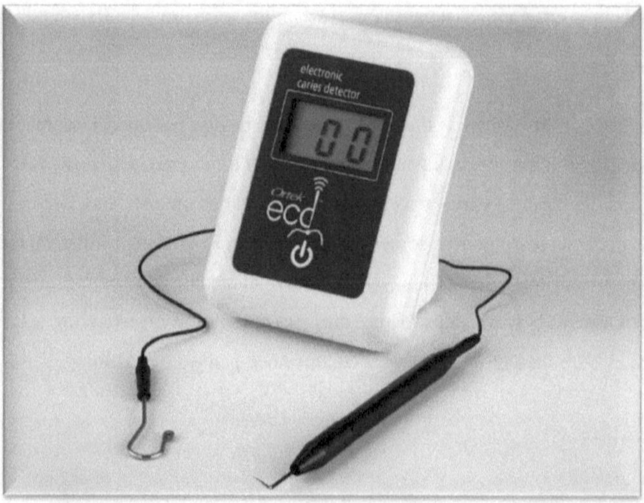

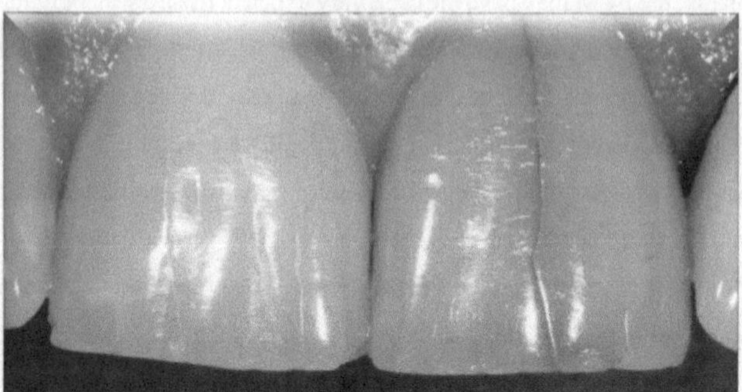

3.11 Electrical impedance tomography (EIT)

Experimental methods for caries diagnosis, which rely on measuring electrical conductance, typically employ a two-point measurement setup. This approach necessitates the probe electrode to be in direct contact with the actual site of the lesion. However, since these measurements are confined to specific discrete locations, their selection is primarily guided by visual cues indicating carious involvement. Consequently, electrical conductance measurements conducted in this manner are deemed unreliable.

Even when the tooth surface is covered by a conducting medium, allowing for surface-specific measurements without direct tooth contact, there has been no observed increase in test sensitivity. This lack of improvement is attributed to the expanded measurement area and variations in occlusal surfaces among individual teeth, resulting in differences in electrode contact area. Additionally, factors such as probe pressure and minor temperature fluctuations can influence the measurements.[39]

A significant impetus for developing methods like Electrical Impedance Tomography (EIT) stems from the morphology of caries itself, particularly the presence of a remineralized surface layer that encases the actual lesion, thereby electrically insulating the electrode contact. Thus, an alternative configuration is warranted, one where diagnostic interpretation no longer relies on quantitative parameters.

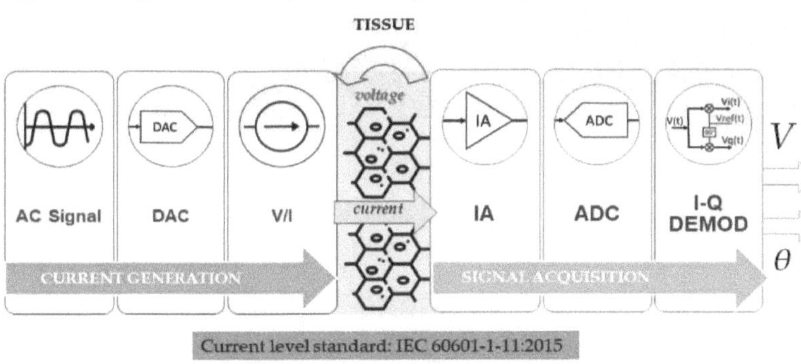

3.12 Laser

Laser fluorescence for detecting caries was first showcased in the early 1980s. Since then, researchers have refined the technique, highlighting distinctions in the fluorescent light emitted from healthy and carious tooth surfaces. Typically, these variations are captured using a digital camera and presented on a computer monitor.[42]

The scientific principle underlying this method is that when enamel is illuminated with blue light from an Argon laser, it emits yellow light through autofluorescence. However, in the presence of caries, the intensity of this fluorescence diminishes. This reduction occurs due to light scattering within the lesion.[43]

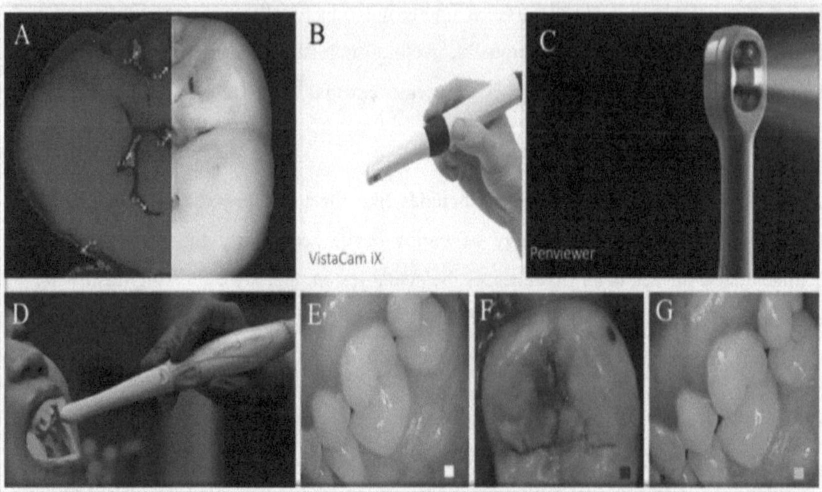

3.13 Quantitative light-induced fluorescence (QLF)

Differences in fluorescence are analysed using specialized software (QLF-Quantitative Laser Fluorescence), where areas of darker Gray enamel under illumination indicate early (incipient) caries. Some experiments have employed a fluorescent dye to potentially enhance this effect. However, as of now, no additional benefit has been observed with the dye technique.[44,45]

Another group of researchers has explored using filtered visible white light instead of a laser as the light source for fluorescence, aiming to eliminate the need for a laser. This filtered white light technique, analysed through a clinical camera, demonstrates comparable results to those obtained with an argon laser.[46-48]

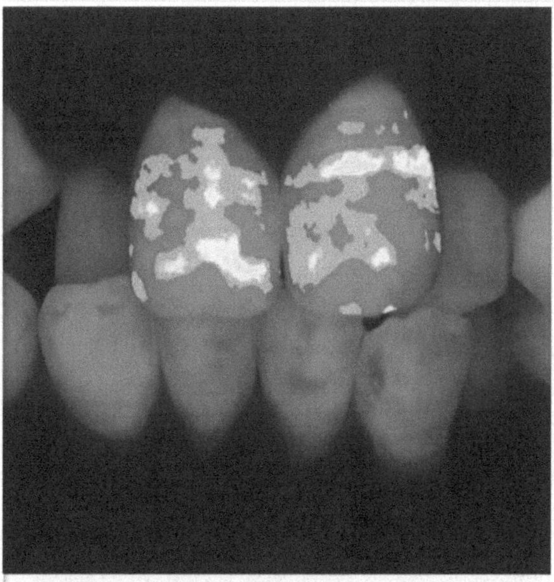

Quantitative Light Fluorescence (QLF) and Polarized White Light (PWL) assessments of dental fluorosis in an epidemiological setting

3.14 Infrared Laser Fluorescence (DIAGNOdent®)

A compact handheld device, DIAGNOdent (KaVo Dental, Germany), has recently been introduced to the market. Unlike traditional methods that use blue light, this device utilizes red light with a wavelength of 655nm and an output of less than 1mW. The red laser light identifies caries by detecting increased fluorescence in affected areas compared to sound tooth structure. In contrast, blue light highlights caries by revealing reduced fluorescence in affected areas.[49]

These differences stem from the distinct characteristics of light at different wavelengths and their effects on teeth and caries lesions. The phenomenon appears to be driven by the enhanced fluorescence of cariogenic bacterial metabolites within the lesion, along with changes in the lesion's fluorescent properties.[50]

The Diagnodent unit from KaVo is designed as a pen-like device with detachable tips of varying diameters. Its core features a red laser Fiber, with surrounding Fibers serving as detectors to measure the fluorescent light reflected from the tooth surface. The device provides readings on a digital display accompanied by an audible tone, with higher readings and pitch indicating a greater likelihood of caries involvement, particularly at the amelodentinal junction and underlying dentin. Each patient requires individual calibration, typically by setting a baseline level on a healthy tooth. While no definitive value indicates the presence of caries or the need for intervention, scores above 25 suggest a high probability of caries.[51]

The device enables monitoring without the need for exploratory cavity preparation or radiographs. However, its optimal performance is observed on smooth surfaces and in occlusal pits and fissures. Limitations include the requirement for clean and dry tooth surfaces and fissures during assessment. To date, there is no evidence supporting the use of Diagnodent for detecting approximal or secondary caries adjacent to existing restorations, let alone recurrent caries beneath restorations, whether metallic or tooth-coloured. The presence of existing restorations or fissure sealants may affect the accuracy of the device.[51]

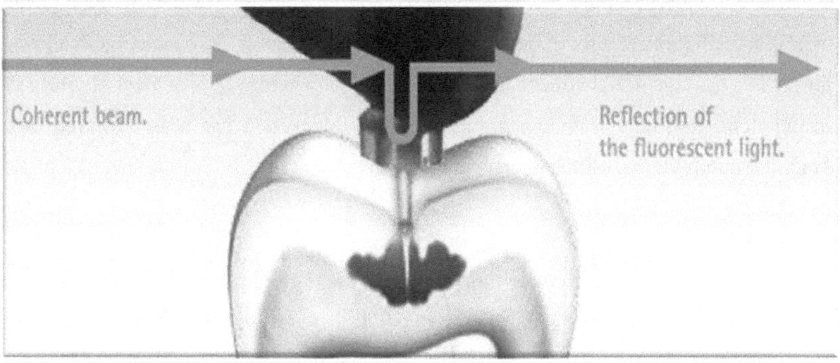

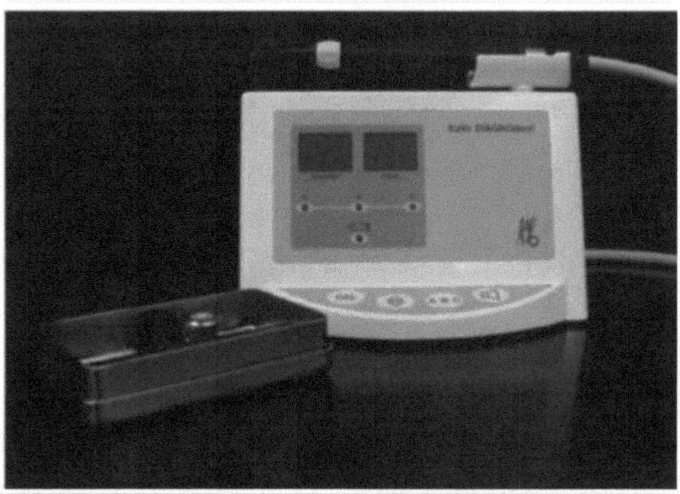

3.15 Fibre Optic Transillumination (FOTI)

FOTI presents an alternative diagnostic approach that can complement clinical examination. Most practitioners are familiar with the method of using a bright Fiber optic light to transilluminate a tooth, revealing the presence of caries. The intact tooth allows for the free passage of light due to minimal absorption, whereas carious areas absorb and scatter light, resulting in darkened appearances. However, it has been observed that examiner interpretation of this phenomenon varies.[52]

Newer iterations of this technique utilize digital imaging Fiber optic transillumination, where the transient light image is captured by a digital camera. This allows for a more precise assessment of caries shadows. Studies have demonstrated that this method is significantly more sensitive in detecting early lesions compared to radiographs. Furthermore, the procedure has been histologically validated and exhibits sensitivity and specificity levels surpassing those of radiographs.[53]

Given its computer-based nature and the indication of good reproducibility in results, this technology enables accurate monitoring of lesion development. This progress in technology since the 1980s, when a study involving 3000 children in Scotland found bitewing radiographs to be notably more accurate in detecting early approximal lesions, highlights the advancement in this field.[54]

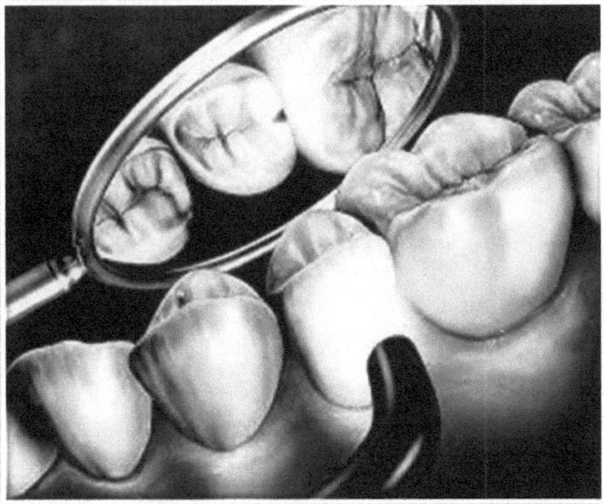

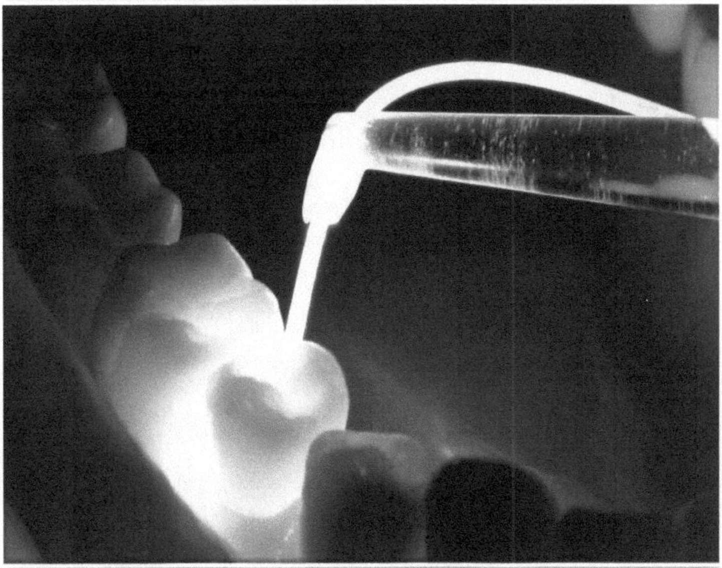

3.16 Alternating Current Impedance Spectroscopy Technique

The Alternating Current Impedance Spectroscopy Technique (ACIST) is utilized to characterize the electrical properties of both a tooth and its lesion, facilitating the monitoring and quantification of changes over time. When applying alternating current to a tooth immersed in saliva, an ionic current flow is generated, with a mean value of zero, which does not polarize the electrolyte solution. Electrical impedance measurements not only reflect resistance but also consider other factors that impede current flow.[55]

When electrical impedance spectroscopy is employed to characterize dental hard tissues containing ionic pores, it measures ion movement, with these measurements indicating the current size of the pores. In carious dental tissues, the pores are typically larger compared to sound tissue. A clinical study focusing on root caries tested this method, concluding that repeated measurements over time could indicate changes in pore size, hence signalling whether caries is progressing or regressing.[55]

Although smaller pore sizes were associated with greater resistance (impedance) measurements, there was some overlap among experimental groups. Further refinement and validation of this technique are necessary to establish it as a potential tool for diagnosing and monitoring caries progression over time.[55]

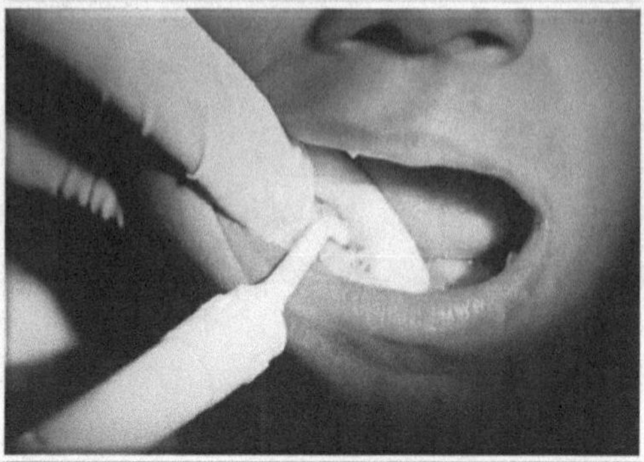

3.17 Microbial Testing

Recent evaluations of microbial tests, such as S. mutans and Lactobacillus sp. counts, for diagnosing and predicting caries activity have determined that while these tests have some utility, they are most effective when used alongside other diagnostic methods for individual patients. They are particularly valuable when initially measured to establish a baseline value for the patient, and then periodically monitored to detect any changes indicative of increased caries risk. However, limitations in the accuracy of these tests may persist despite further research efforts, owing to the inherent biology of these organisms and their interactions with the individual host.[56]

Verdenshocht and colleagues examined advancements in caries diagnosis and their implications for treatment decisions. In the past, when caries prevalence was higher, visual inspection and radiographic examination were sufficient for diagnosing caries requiring operative treatment. However, with declining caries prevalence, these methods are no longer suitable for all patients. For most patients in Western countries, caries detection now focuses on identifying small lesions.[56]

Their meta-analysis on diagnostic tests for occlusal caries revealed that visual inspection performed poorly, while electrical conductivity methods performed the best. Similarly, their analysis for approximal caries indicated that radiography outperformed Fiber-optic transillumination. When histologic lesion depth or mineral loss was used for validation, quantitative Fiber-optic transillumination showed the highest correlation with lesion depth for approximal lesions, while visual inspection based on translucency and enamel breakdown on air drying performed best for occlusal surfaces, followed by electrical conductivity methods.[56]

Verdenshocht and colleagues highlighted a study demonstrating that clinicians can enhance their performance by using a detailed scoring system and ensuring thorough examination after drying the field. Quantitative methods showed the highest correlation with lesion depth and have the potential to monitor small changes over time.[56]

Given that caries is a chronic, slowly progressive disease, its effects may not be detected until years after onset. Early detection of caries signs in young patients is time-consuming, and it is more beneficial to focus on identifying early signs of caries in high-risk patients. Assessing a patient's caries risk should involve a comprehensive evaluation of all pertinent factors contributing to caries etiology, such as diet, saliva flow, and cariogenic microbes. Verdenshocht and colleagues demonstrated that caries-related factors, such as DMFS, DMFT, and caries in first molars, were the most reliable predictors of future caries onset. However, combinations of multiple caries prediction tests performed less accurately than existing caries as a predictor.[56]

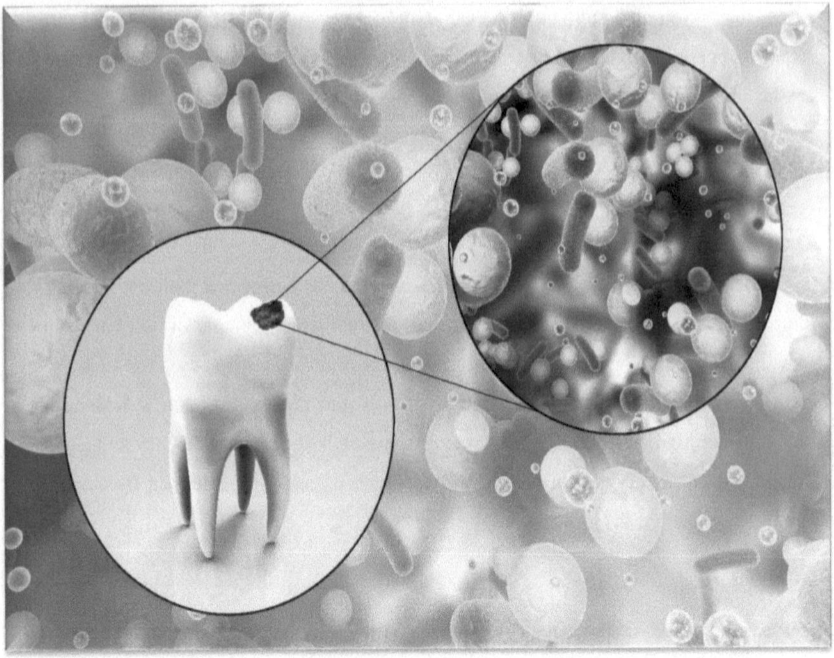

3.18 Magnetic resonance micro-imagery

This method utilizes a controlled magnetic field akin to MRI. In laboratory settings, it has demonstrated the capability to generate precise three-dimensional reconstructions of teeth and caries lesions, confirmed by histological examinations. Regrettably, this technology is not yet accessible for clinical use. MRM shows promise for investigating the progression of dental caries, particularly when employed in conjunction with other techniques.[57]

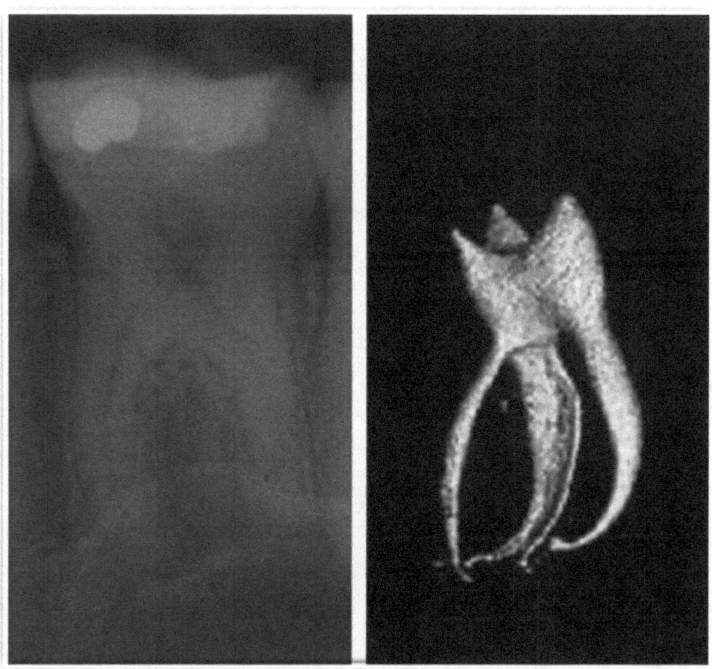

3.19 Caries-Detecting Dyes

In 1972, a technique utilizing a red basic fuchsin stain was proposed (and subsequently refined) to assist in distinguishing between the two layers of carious dentin.[58] Due to potential carcinogenic properties, the basic fuchsin stain was later substituted with another dye, acid red solution. Since then, several protein dyes have been introduced as agents for caries detection.[59] Designed to facilitate the complete removal of infected carious dentin while minimizing the removal of sound dentin, these dyes were claimed to selectively stain only infected tissue, promoting a "pain-free" caries removal technique without the need for local anesthesia. However, the technique was labour-intensive, relying on staining guidance, multiple applications and removals of dye, and the use of a slow-speed bur.[60]

Traditionally, tactile and visual assessments are employed to determine the absence of caries in a cavity, making the idea of a diagnostic aid capable of distinguishing infected dentin appealing. Subsequent clinical trials were conducted in the United States and the United Kingdom involving the application of the dye in cavities prepared by dental students, which were deemed caries-free by their clinical instructors. These trials revealed dye-stained dentin at the enamel–dentin junction in 57% to 59% of cavities. This suggested that the clinical judgment of the instructors was often flawed and indicated a high prevalence of residual decay.[61] However, it's worth noting that the UK study's laboratory component did not link dye-stained material with infection but rather with lower levels of mineralization, with or without infection. Notably, all authors expressed particular concern regarding the amelo-dentinal junction. Moreover, the researchers deemed dye staining on more than 50% of the cavity pulpal floors, as judged complete by instructors, inappropriate for further dentin removal, as it could lead to unnecessary pulpal exposures.[62]

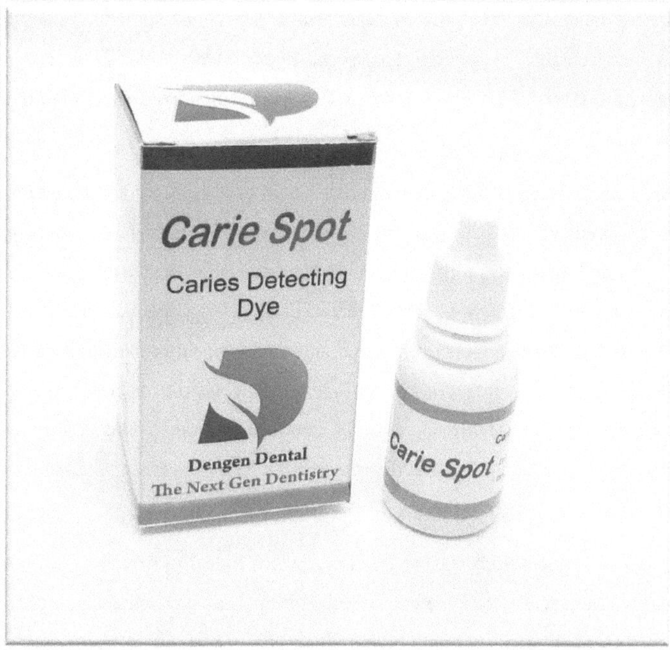
Carie Spot
Caries Detecting
Dye
Dengen Dental
The Next Gen Dentistry
Carie Spot

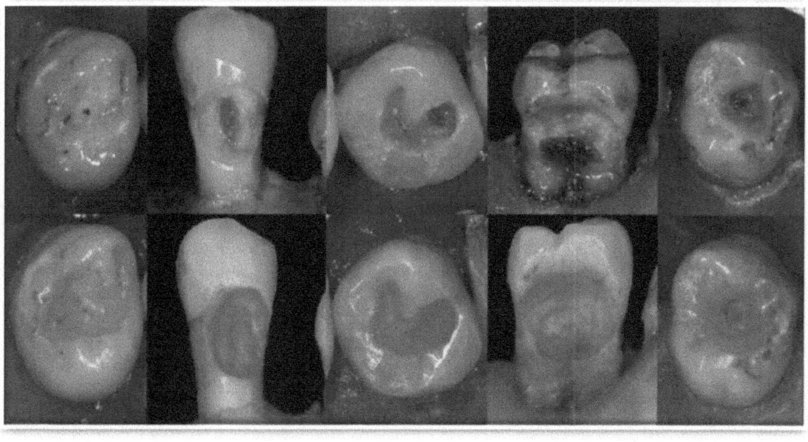

Use of Caries-Detector Dyes for Occlusal Caries :-

The efficacy of utilizing dyes for detecting carious enamel has raised significant doubts. For instance, many dyes, like procion dyes, lead to permanent staining, rendering them clinically unacceptable. Although fluorescent dyes' intensity has been observed to correlate with mineral loss, they are only specific to demineralization, similar to dentinal caries-detector dyes.[63]

Electronic caries detectors have shown reliability in predicting dentin demineralization beneath non-cavitated enamel. However, subsequent dentin samples in such cases often indicate minimal or no bacterial infection. Neither visual inspection nor electronic readings consistently identify heavily infected dentin. Bitewing radiographic analysis emerged as the most dependable diagnostic method. Studies have indicated low bacterial counts in radiographically intact fissures, whereas lesions visible in dentin on radiographs are associated with a notable increase in dentin infection.[64] This underscores the appropriateness of managing affected susceptible fissures through fissure sealing, especially when they appear radiographically sound.

Lussi et al. conducted a study focusing on Diagnodent for caries detection and concluded that it serves as a valuable complement to clinical examination. Their analysis of available data suggests that Diagnodent exhibits reproducibility in caries detection, demonstrating good sensitivity and specificity, particularly at the D2 and D3 levels. The method is most effective for detecting caries on occlusal and easily accessible smooth surfaces. The observed reproducibility allows for longitudinal monitoring of the caries process and assessment of preventive measures' outcomes, provided Diagnodent is combined with a positioning system. However, false-positive readings may occur due to fluorescence from materials or molecules.[65]

Additionally, **Peker et al.** evaluated the effectiveness of operating microscopes compared to unaided visual examination, conventional, and digital intraoral radiography for detecting proximal caries. Their findings suggest that the efficiency of the operating microscope is statistically equivalent to unaided visual examination but lower than radiographic systems for proximal caries detection.[65]

CONCEPTS & DEPENDENCY

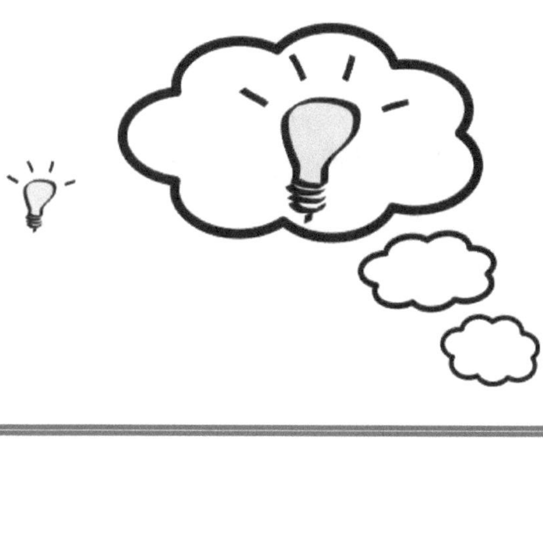

The three main concepts of MID are:

A. Identification
B. Prevention
C. Control

Identification:

- Caries Activity Tests
- Saliva Analysis

Prevention:

- Diet analysis and counselling.
- Use of sugar substitutes.
- Combating Microorganisms (Chlorhexidine, Triclosan).
- Increase the Resistance of teeth to decay.
- Fluorides, Pit and sealants, Laser.

Control:

- Preventive Resin Restoration
- Atraumatic Restorative Treatment

4.1 Identification

Identification of Caries:

- Caries activity tests
- Saliva analysis

Caries activity tests:

Caries activity denotes the increase in active lesions, including new and recurrent ones, observed over a specified period. It serves as a gauge of the pace at which a carious lesion advances.

The advantages of caries activity tests include:

1. Enhanced comprehension of caries progression.
2. Identification of individuals with a higher likelihood of developing caries.
3. Provision of customized preventive programs for patients before extensive dental restorative procedures are undertaken.

Several caries activity tests exist, including the Lactobacillus colony count test, Calorimetric Snyder test, swab test, Streptococcus mutans level in saliva assessment, dip slide method for S. mutans count, salivary buffer capacity test, enamel solubility test, salivary reductase test, Alban test, Streptococcus mutans screening test, and Fosdick calcium dissolution test.

However, these tests have limitations. None are highly reliable in predicting caries increments, which is unsurprising as they typically measure single parameters such as acid production or bacterial colony counts. Dental caries is a multifactorial disease, and caries predictive tests do not encompass factors affecting caries resistance, such as fluoride exposure, enamel maturation, or immune protection.

Saliva Analysis:

Saliva analysis can yield vital insights into secretion rates, buffering capacity, and the presence of streptococcus mutans and lactobacilli. While bacterial counts may aid in assessing populations, they might not provide accurate information for individual patients. However, understanding the significance of high colony-forming unit (CFU) values can help identify high-risk patients. Salivary pH tests can be conducted using pH paper.

The **DENTOBUFF METHOD** (Orion Diagnostica, Espoo, Finland) offers a convenient way to measure saliva's buffer capacity. This dip-slide technique involves impregnating dip-sticks with chemical indicators instead of agar gel.

The **dip-sticks** are then immersed or coated with the patient's whole saliva, producing a color indicative of the saliva's ability to buffer acids and bases.

Saliva's buffer capacity serves as the most reliable indicator of caries activity. Caries disease begins long before cavities form, often due to factors like increased sugar consumption, frequent eating, or a decline in protective saliva properties. These changes can be gauged using chair-side tests for saliva buffering capacity, pH, viscosity, and flow, as well as tests for oral bacteria levels.

4.2 Prevention

Preventive treatment methods aim to minimize tooth demineralization caused by cariogenic bacteria, thereby preventing cavitated lesions. These methods include:

1. Limiting pathogen growth and metabolism.
2. Increasing the resistance of the tooth surface to demineralization.

Prevention Methods:

A. Diet analysis and counselling:

Understanding the relationship between diet and caries prevalence requires gathering information about food consumption and dietary habits.

Various methods for data collection include :-

- Food balance sheets.
- Food accounts.
- Estimated food records.
- Weighing methods.
- Duplicate portion technique.
- Interviews.
- Questionnaires.

B. Sugar substitutes:

Artificial sweeteners approved by the FDA, such as aspartame, saccharin, acesulfame-K, neotame, tagatose, and sucralose, can help reduce calorie intake, manage conditions like diabetes, and potentially prevent cavities.

C. Combating microorganisms:

Chlorhexidine operates by diminishing the population of cariogenic bacteria due to its broad spectrum of activity against both Gram-positive and Gram-negative bacteria. Its unique attribute of being bacteriostatic at low concentrations and bactericidal at higher concentrations positions it as the 'Gold standard'. Upon rinsing with a 0.2% chlorhexidine solution, there is an immediate decrease in salivary bacterial counts. This reduction endures for several hours owing to the substantivity of chlorhexidine within saliva and on tooth surfaces.

For individuals at high risk for caries, Maxwell H. Anderson et al have recommended a regimen of rinsing with 0.2% chlorhexidine for two weeks once every 3-4 months. This regimen has been claimed to be effective against Streptococcus mutans and lactobacilli. When followed by twice-daily fluoride mouth rinses and the use of fluoride toothpaste, a synergistic effect is observed. Additionally, 40% chlorhexidine varnishes are available, and Emilson et al found them to be superior and more effective than chlorhexidine rinses, gels, and even fluoride varnishes.

Long-term application of combinations of amine/stannous fluoride or Triclosan/additive, such as triclosan copolymer, has been suggested as plaque control agents by Zimmermann et al (1992), Conforti et al (1994), Hickel (1997), and Schiffner (2000).

D. Increasing the resistance of teeth to decay:

Fluoride plays a significant role in the demineralization-remineralization cycle. When demineralization occurs in the presence of free fluoride ions, the remineralization process is facilitated, resulting in the deposition of fluorapatite instead of hydroxyapatite within the lesion's surface.

E. Pit & Fissure Sealants:

Why are sealants essential?

Due to their structure, pit and fissure surfaces are often challenging to clean, increasing the risk of caries. Even a single bristle from a toothbrush is too large to effectively clean these fissures. Furthermore, pits and fissures are less susceptible to the protective effects of fluoride compared to smooth enamel surfaces, as evidenced by research.

Efficacy of Sealants : -

Pit and fissure sealants were introduced to the dental profession in 1967, and their efficacy was acknowledged by the ADA in 1971. Presently, the ADA's Council on Scientific Affairs has approved ten different sealant materials.

F. Lasers in caries prevention:

The use of lasers in preventing caries has been under investigation since the 1960s. Adrian, in 1977, reported initial findings on the effects of pulsed Nd: YAG laser on dental pulps in monkeys, comparing them with the ruby laser. Various types of lasers have been studied, including ruby, Nd: YAG, CO_2, and argon lasers. Some researchers aimed to enhance resistance to caries by reducing demineralization rates of enamel and dentin, while others explored alternative treatments for sealing pits and fissures.[66]

4.3 Control

There are two elements to the biological approach.

1. Alteration of the oral environment in order to minimize demineralization.
2. Application of agents such as chlorhexidine and topical fluoride.

Alteration of Oral environment is brought by:

- Reduced frequency of refined carbohydrate intake.
- Optimum Plaque control.
- Optimum Salivary flow
- Patient education.
- Preventive resin restoration
- Atraumatic Restorative Technique

Preventive Resin Restoration:

The Preventive Resin Restoration represents a natural progression from the use of occlusal sealants. It combines the preventive principles of sealant therapy for caries in vulnerable pits and fissures with the therapeutic aspect of restoring incipient caries using composite resin on the same occlusal surface. This technique offers the most conservative approach to addressing confined, early-stage occlusal caries in young permanent teeth. It involves minimal tooth preparation while ensuring future caries prevention through sealant application. By placing resin in the carious areas and adjacent susceptible regions, it seals them off from the oral environment. This approach serves as a valuable treatment option, offering an alternative to traditional restorations like amalgam.[13]

Benefits of PRR:

- Requires minimal cavity preparation, preserving healthy tooth structure and retention.
- Halts tooth destruction by sealing caries, particularly effective for teeth with pits and fissures.
- Reduces the risk of microleakage.
- Offers less invasive restoration replacement compared to conventional methods like amalgam.[13]

Atraumatic Restorative Treatment (ART):

The acronym ART stands for Atraumatic Restorative Treatment, an approach for dental caries management. It involves the gentle removal of soft, demineralized tooth tissue using manual instruments, followed by restoration with an adhesive material, typically glass ionomer. This treatment method is endorsed by the World Health Organization to extend restorative dental care to underserved populations who lack access to traditional dental services. ART was developed as an alternative to extraction in disadvantaged areas, aiming to preserve as many teeth as possible and significantly contributes to achieving universal dental health goals.[67]

Advantages of ART:

1. Simplicity
2. Good patient acceptance, especially by children.
3. Local anesthetics and dental hand pieces are usually not required.
4. Minimal surgical intervention.
5. Conservation of sound tooth structure.
6. Reduced risk for subsequent endodontics and tooth extraction.
7. Increased survival time of the affected teeth.
8. Dental equipment is not needed, nor electricity.
9. Infection control is relatively simple as only a small set of hand instruments are used.

Disadvantages:

1. Can be fatigue of preparing the cavities with hand instruments.
2. Increases the chances of leaving residual caries.
3. Requirements for accurately handling the material.
4. Inadequate strength of the filling materials to resist occlusal forces.
5. Loss of restorations from shallow and non-macro mechanically retentive preparation.

Dependency

M.I.D depends on :-

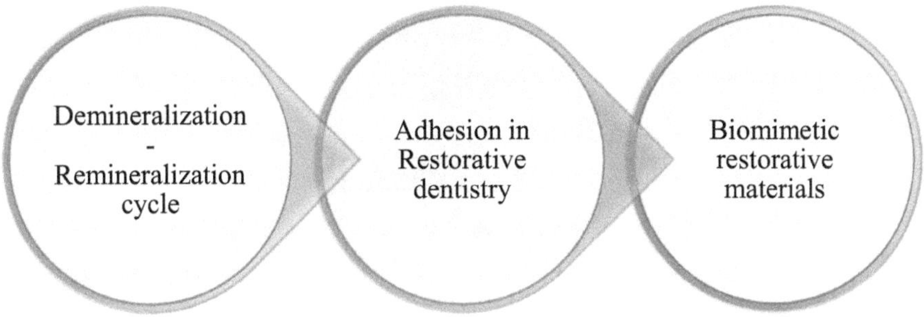

Demineralization-Remineralization cycle

Caries is a complex bacterial infection characterized by a cycle of demineralization and remineralization, primarily driven by the activity of Streptococcus mutans and Lactobacilli in dental plaque. Following removal through brushing or prophylaxis, dental plaque quickly re-forms on the pellicle layer. Within hours of formation, cariogenic bacteria populate the plaque, with a shift in bacterial composition as plaque matures.[68] Demineralization occurs when these bacteria produce acids that erode tooth enamel, resulting in mineral loss. This process is initiated by the metabolism of fermentable carbohydrates, leading to acid production and pH reduction. Remineralization, crucially dependent on factors like saliva and mineral ions, can counteract demineralization.

In the initial stages, demineralization targets the enamel, causing calcium and phosphate ion depletion. Repeated demineralization without adequate remineralization can lead to the formation of visible carious lesions, often appearing as white spots.[69] These lesions signify decalcification with subsurface dissolution, initially preserving the tooth's surface integrity. It's suggested that fluoride and salivary proteins may mitigate surface dissolution by adsorbing onto enamel crystals. White spots are frequently observed in teenagers undergoing orthodontic treatment with fixed appliances, attributed to challenges in plaque control around bands and patient compliance.[70] Typically, white spots may exhibit a rough texture when gently explored with a dental instrument.

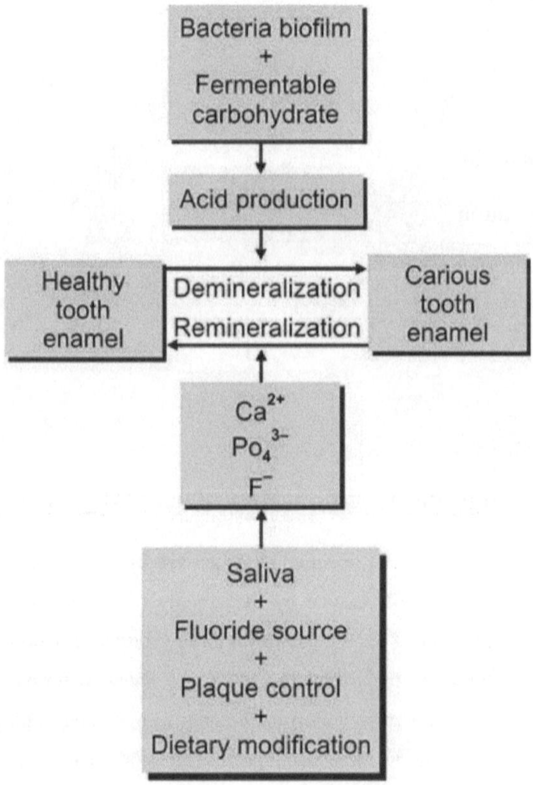

Natural Reversal of Demineralization

Saliva serves as a natural remedy for demineralization, containing essential calcium and phosphate ions, along with buffering agents, fluoride, and other compounds. Typically maintaining a pH range of 6.8 to 7 in healthy individuals, saliva effectively counteracts decreases in pH on tooth surfaces.[17] However, as acidity levels rise and persist, saliva's buffering capacity diminishes, hindering remineralization efforts. In instances where demineralization outweighs remineralization, lesions may develop. During the early stages of lesion formation, changes may not be visible, but in cases of white spot lesions, they can progress to an enamel surface that appears frosty, yet feels hard and smooth to the touch. Remineralization initiates as pH levels increase, allowing calcium, phosphate, and fluoride from saliva to infiltrate and repair the subsurface lesion, resulting in a more resilient layer compared to the original enamel.[71]

Understanding and applying this knowledge in practice are crucial for improving dental health. This involves conducting risk assessments, preventing and halting caries progression, promoting natural repair processes, and embracing minimally invasive dental techniques.

PRINCIPLES

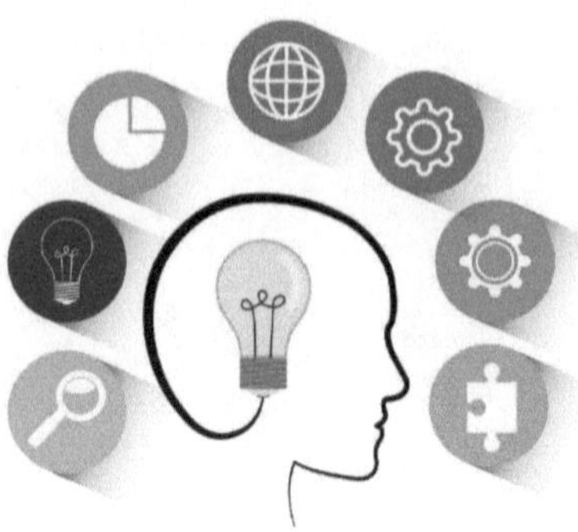

1. Early caries diagnosis.
2. Classification of caries depth and progression.
3. Remineralization of early lesions.
4. Minimal surgical intervention of caries lesions.
5. Repair rather than a replacement of defective restoration.
6. Assess disease management outcomes at intervals.

3.1 Early caries diagnosis

In children, prior to the onset of cavitation, dental caries begins due to exposure to risk factors like increased sugar consumption, frequent eating, or changes in the protective properties of saliva. These alterations can be assessed through chair-side tests, including the evaluation of saliva quality, quantity, pH, buffering capacity, and oral bacterial levels.

Initial carious lesions represent primary stages before cavitation occurs. Visual examination is crucial to detect changes in enamel colour, translucency, and structure. Wet surface inspection can reveal cavities, as well as brown or white stains, tooth by tooth. Additionally, initial assessments may include checking periodontal status and existing restorations. Evaluating caries activity involves observing plaque buildup and gingival pathology in suspect areas. A blunt or rounded probe, applied gently, can assess tactile perceptions and the gingival margin's status regarding bleeding upon probing. Extensive clinical observation notes changes in colour and translucency indicative of demineralization.

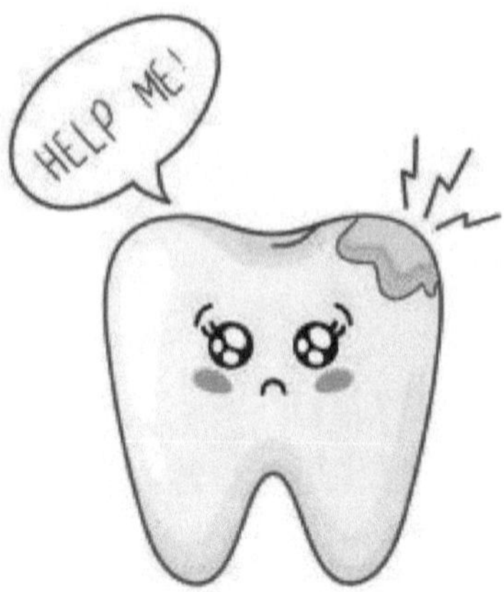

These visual cues are categorized in systems like the International Caries Detection and Assessment System (ICDAS), featuring six codes. Initial lesions predominantly fall under Codes 1 and 2:

- ICDAS II Code 0: Indicates a healthy tooth.
- ICDAS II Code 1: First visible changes in the enamel. Visible only after drying with air. Changes in coloration confined to areas of pits.
- ICDAS II Code 2: Change in visible enamel even in the presence of moisture. More extensive and not restricted to pits.
- ICDAS II Code 3: Destruction located in enamel without visible dentin, discontinuities of enamel surface.
- ICDAS II Code 4: Dark shadow on the underlying dentin, with or without localized destruction of enamel.
- ICDAS II Code 5: Clear cavity with visible dentin; cavity that involves less than half the dental surface cavity that involves less than half the dental surface.
- ICDAS II Code 6: Extensive cavity evident in dentin; cavity deep and wide, involves more than half of the tooth.

New diagnostic aids, such as electrical conductance measurement, quantitative light-induced fluorescence, dye-enhanced laser fluorescence, Diagnodent, Fiber optic transillumination, digital radiology, digital subtraction radiography, optical coherence tomography, and tuned aperture computed tomography, offer early caries detection capabilities.[2,4]

ICDAS II

Score 0	Score 1	Score 2	Score 3	Score 4	Score 5	Score 6
No visual signs of carious lesions or any enamel defect	First visible changes in the enamel. Visible only after drying with air. Changes in coloration confined to areas of pits	Change in visible enamel even in the presence of moisture. More extensive and not restricted to pits.	Destruction located in enamel without visible dentin, discontinuities of enamel surface	Dark shadow on the underlying dentin, with or without localized destruction of enamel	Clear cavity with visible dentin; cavity that involves less than half the dental surface	Extensive cavity evident in dentin; cavity deep and wide, involves more than half of the tooth

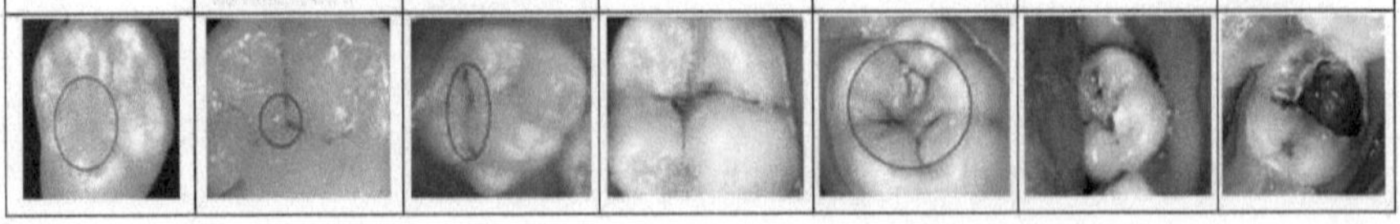

ICDAS II system have two digit coding for detection criteria of primary coronal caries. The first one is related to the restoration of teeth and has a coding that ranges from 0 to 9. The second digit ranges from 0 to 6 that is used for coding the caries. There are minor variations between the visual signs associated with each code depending on a number of factors. Therefore; a detailed description of each of the codes is given under the following headings: Pits and fissures, smooth surface (mesial or distal), free smooth surfaces and caries associated with restorations and sealants (CARS).

0	Surface not restored or sealed	5	Stainless steel crown
1	Sealant, partial	6	Porcelain or gold or PFM crown or veneer
2	Sealant, full	7	Lost or broken restoration
3	Tooth colored restoration	8	Temporary restoration
4	Amalgam restoration	9	Used for the following conditions:
			96:Tooth surface cannot be examined
			97: Tooth missing because of caries
			98: Tooth missing for reasons other than caries
			99: Unerupted

3.2 Classification of Caries depth and progression

Recently, a novel classification has been proposed, urging the dental profession to reconsider operative dentistry through a fresh perspective. Despite the challenging oral conditions, there exist restorative materials that exhibit enduring adhesion to tooth structure, encompassing both enamel and dentin. Additionally, there have been advancements in cavity preparation instruments. Consequently, it has been recommended that the profession embrace new classification systems, which take into account the location and extent of lesions, along with radiographic assessments.[5]

Classification based on site and size of the lesion

In response to the importance of site and size of carious lesions for treatment, Mount and colleagues have proposed a new classification, which classifies lesions by combining both their site and size. This is reflected in a dual coding system and is expressed in the form of a grid.[6]

Firstly, lesions are classified according to their location:

- Site 1: pits and fissures (occlusal and other smooth tooth surfaces);
- Site 2: contact area between two teeth;
- Site 3: cervical area in contact with gingival tissues.

		Size				
		No cavity 0	Minimal 1	Moderate 2	Enlarged 3	Extensive 4
	Pit/fissure 1	1.0	1.1	1.2	1.3	1.4
Site	Contact area 2	2.0	2.1	2.2	2.3	2.4
	Cervical 3	3.0	3.1	3.2	3.3	3.4

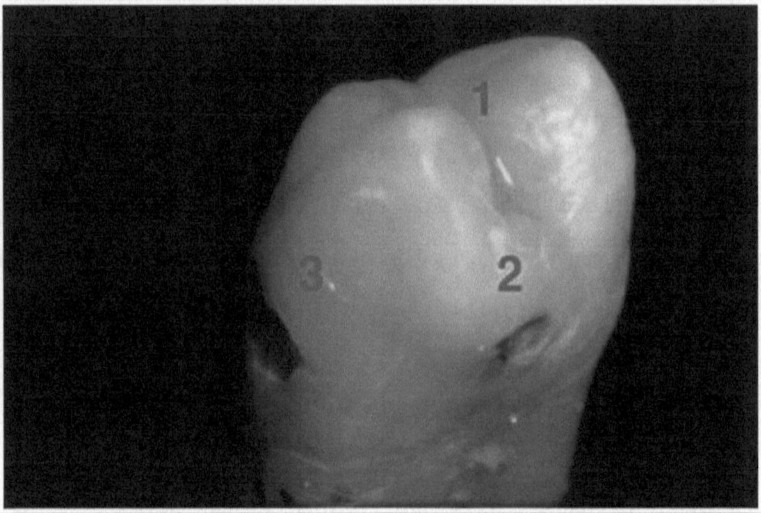

Secondly, the new classification identifies carious lesions according to various sizes:

- Size 0: carious lesion without cavitation can be remineralized.
- Size 1: small cavitation, just beyond healing through remineralization.
- Size 2: moderate cavity not extended to cusps.
- Size 3: enlarged cavity, with at least one cusp which is undermined and which needs protection from occlusal load.
- Size 4: extensive cavity, with at least one lost cusp or incisal edge.

A direct comparison between the standard GV Black classification and the new classification which is recommended for modern operative dentistry.	
New Classification	**GV Black Classification**
Site 1 – Pits, Fissures And Smooth Surfaces.	**Class I – Pits & fissures**
Size 0 – Fissure seal.	Not classified
Size 1 – Minimal surgery.	Not classified
Size 2 – Equivalent to black class 1.	Class I
Size 3 – Requires protection for maintaining tooth structure.	Class I
Size 4 – Lost cusp or similar.	Class I
Site 2 – Contact Area, All Teeth **Size 0** – Surface demineralisation. **Size I** – Beyond remineralisation. **Size 2** – Moderate involvement. **Size 3** – Requires protection of remaining tooth structure. **Size 4** – Bulk loss of tooth structure.	**Class II – Contact area, Posteriors** Not classified Not classified Class II Class II Class II **Class III – Contact area, Anteriors** Not classified Not classified Class III Not classified **Class IV – Incisal edge lost, Anteriors** Not classified Not classified Not classified Class IV
Site 3 – Cervical Third	**Class V – Cervical Third**
Size 0 – Surface demineralisation	Not classified
Size 1 – Minimal intervention	Not classified
Size 2 – More extensive	Class V
Size 3 – Approximal root surface	Class II
Size 4 – Two or more surfaces	Class II

Radiographic evaluation of proximal caries

Early proximal lesions are defined as radiolucencies detected in the inner half of enamel, at the dentinoenamel junction (DEJ), or even slightly penetrating into the dentin, yet displaying minimal or no cavitation. These radiographic changes in proximal lesions can be evaluated using the classification proposed by Ben and Dankel et al.,[2] which includes:

- E1 = Radiolucency in the outer half of enamel.
- E2 = Radiolucency in the inner half of enamel.
- D1 = Radiolucency in the outer third of dentin.
- D2 = Radiolucency in the middle third of dentin.
- D3 = Radiolucency in the inner third of dentin.

Research has indicated that a significant percentage (60% - 80%) of initial proximal lesions with radiolucencies in the outer third of dentin do not progress to cavitation. Therefore, restorative intervention is recommended only when the radiolucent lesion has extended to the D2 region, where the likelihood of cavitation ranges from 20% to 40%.

In managing caries, it is recommended to adhere to these procedural steps in the contemporary approach to treatment.[2]

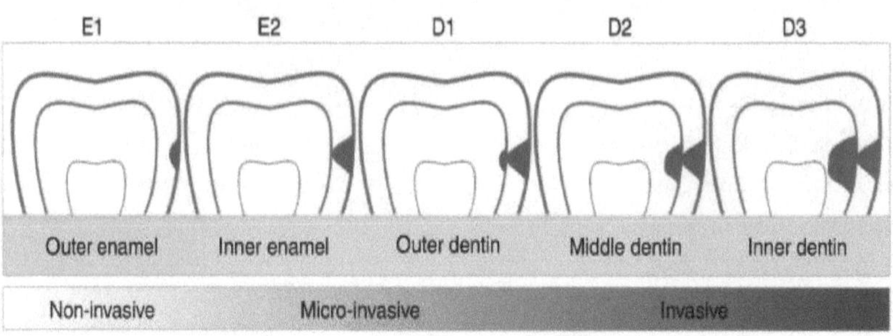

3.3 Remineralization of early lesions

Delivery methods for remineralization encompass a variety of materials, including toothpastes, mouth rinses, gels, pastes, chewing gums, lozenges, foods, and beverages. Certain criteria define an ideal remineralization material[16]:

- It should release calcium and phosphate into the subsurface.
- Excessive calcium delivery should be avoided.
- It should not promote calculus formation.
- Effectiveness at acidic pH levels is essential.
- It should enhance saliva's natural remineralizing properties.
- It should offer advantages over fluoride for novel materials.

Saliva - natural reversal of demineralization

It aids in the reversal of demineralization by containing calcium, phosphate ions, buffering agents, fluoride, and other substances. However, successful remineralization depends on maintaining a proper pH balance, as higher acidity levels hinder salivary buffering capacity and may impede remineralization, leading to lesion development.[17]

Fluoride

It plays a crucial role in the remineralization/demineralization cycle by incorporating into the crystalline structure of carbonated hydroxyapatite. This incorporation reduces crystal solubility and increases enamel mineral precipitation rates, primarily through its stability in the crystal lattice and interaction with calcium ions on the crystal surface.[18]

Casein phosphopeptide-amorphous calcium phosphate (CPP-ACP)

It is derived from milk protein and exhibits the unique ability to bind calcium and phosphate ions, stabilizing amorphous calcium phosphate (ACP) in solution. CPP-ACP localizes ACP on the tooth surface, buffering free calcium and phosphate ion activities, maintaining enamel supersaturation, and preventing demineralization while enhancing remineralization. Combining CPP-ACP with fluoride enhances fluoride's anticaries effectiveness synergistically.[19]

Novamin, a bioactive glass compound, releases calcium, phosphorus, sodium, and silicon ions upon contact with water, saliva, or other body fluids, resulting in the formation of new hydroxycarbonate apatite crystals. This mineralized layer is mechanically robust and more resistant to acid.[20]

Enamelon, comprising unstabilized calcium and phosphate salt with sodium fluoride, delivers fluoride alongside soluble calcium and phosphate through its liquid calcium formula. Enamelon toothpaste reduces white spot lesions and aids in enamel remineralization compromised by acidic beverages.[16]

Glass ionomer cements (GIC) are more efficient compared to other materials such as fluoride varnishes and fluoride-releasing sealants. GIC application over white spot lesions provides mechanical protection to weakened enamel and encourages remineralization through continuous fluoride release. Resin-modified GICs infiltrate lesions with resin, preventing further demineralization while boosting remineralization mechanisms with released fluoride ions.[21]

3.4 Minimal surgical intervention of caries lesions

The principles of minimally invasive restoration are as follows[22]:

- Cavity shape is determined by the extent of caries, with each lesion requiring a unique approach (conservative cavity preparation).
- Only demineralized enamel and infected dentine are removed, while affected dentine may be retained.
- Macromechanical retention is unnecessary.
- Adhesive materials enable restoration of undermined enamel cavities.

Preserving tooth structure through minimally invasive cavity preparations is achievable because adhesive materials do not necessitate mechanical retention features. Biomimetic potential, including the release of fluoride, calcium, and phosphate ions, can enhance the remineralization potential of carious lesions. Materials such as glass ionomer cements and composites can be utilized for this purpose.

The introduction of certain technologies has further expanded possibilities for minimal surgical intervention. One such technique, developed in Tanzania in the mid-1980s, is the **Atraumatic Restorative Treatment** (ART), which involves the removal of carious tooth tissues using only hand instruments and restoration of the cavity with a tooth-adhering restorative material. ART restorations exhibit comparable longevity to resin composite or amalgam restorations and offer benefits such as reduced noise, vibration, and the diminished need for local anesthesia.[23]

Another method of caries removal is the **chemo mechanical approach**, which utilizes a gel to aid in mechanical caries removal while exerting a chemical effect on infected dentine. This method relies on the role of sodium hypochlorite in caries removal.[24]

Enamel cavity preparations leverage the support provided by surrounding dentin, making them suitable for amalgam placement and minimizing tooth surface loss, particularly beneficial for children due to its painless nature.

Mini-box or slot type preparations, advocated by Wilson and McLean, involve removing the marginal ridge without including the occlusal pits and fissures, preserving tooth structure while ensuring access to lesions.[25]

Air abrasion, developed by Dr. Robert Black in 1945, offers a non-rotary, pseudo-mechanical technique for conservative cavity preparation, preserving maximal sound tooth structure. Combined with bonded restorations, it facilitates minimal intervention dentistry.[26]

Laser technology has been reported to selectively remove caries while preserving healthy enamel and dentin, with additional benefits such as reducing sensitivity and being well-tolerated by Paediatric patients.[27]

The Hall's technique, a novel method involving the cementation of prefabricated metal crowns over cavitated teeth without removing decomposed carious dentine, shows promise in reducing the treatment burden of cavitated dentine carious lesions, though further research is needed before widespread adoption.[28]

3.5 Repair rather than a replacement of defective restoration

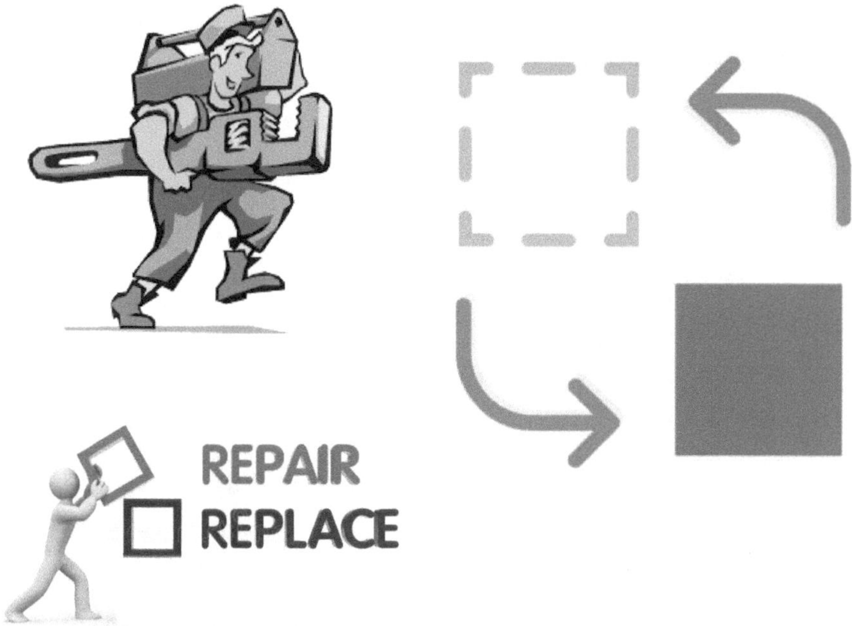

'Replacement dentistry' results in the following consequences:[29]

- Degradation of tooth structure due to the expansion of cavity surface area.
- Complexity in restoration due to the enlarged surface area.
- Larger restorations typically have a shorter lifespan compared to previous ones.
- Risk of potential damage to adjacent teeth.

The decision to repair rather than replace a restoration should always be guided by factors such as the patient's caries risk, the conservative nature of the repair approach, and the professional's assessment of the benefits versus the risks involved.

3.6 Assess disease management outcomes at intervals

Regular follow-up appointments at different intervals are necessary to minimize the likelihood of caries recurrence.

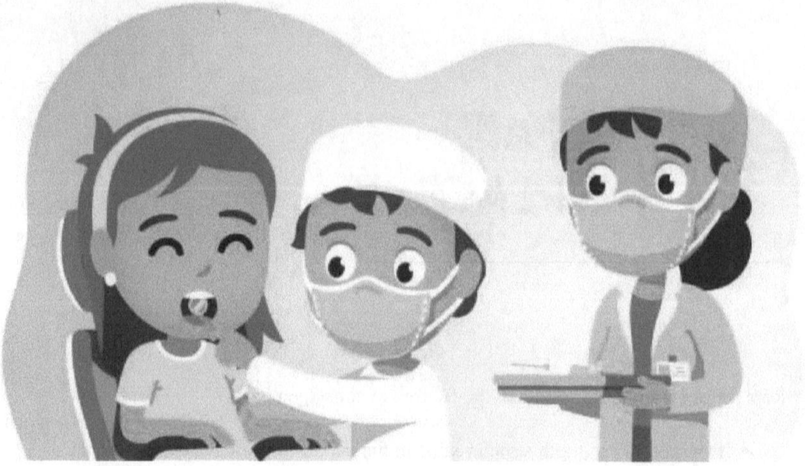

TECHNIQUES

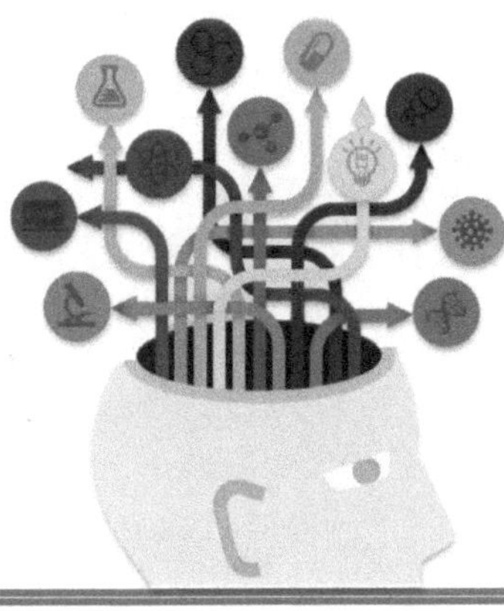

Pit & fissure Sealants	Preventive Resin restorations	Miniature implants versus standard-size implants
Placement of inlays and onlays instead of crowns	Chemo mechanical method of caries removal	ART
Digital radiography versus conventional radiography	Cavity designs for minimal intervention	Lasers
Sonics	Ozone therapy	Genetic modalities in caries prevention
	Enzymes	

6.1 Pit & fissure Sealants

Simenson R.J (1978)[72] provided a definition of pit and fissure sealants as a substance applied into the occlusal pits and fissures of teeth prone to decay, forming a protective layer bonded through micromechanical means. This layer effectively blocks access of caries-producing bacteria to their source of nutrients.

Mathewson (1987)[73] described occlusal sealants as the application and mechanical bonding of a resin material to enamel surfaces etched with acid, thus sealing existing pits and fissures from exposure to the oral environment.

Shobha Tandon (2001)[74] defined fissure sealants as materials applied to occlude pits and fissures primarily found on the occlusal surfaces of molars and premolars. These materials, once applied in fluid form, are polymerized to create a barrier.

A sealant is a transparent or opaque plastic material applied to the pits and fissures of teeth prone to decay. Its primary purpose is to create a physical barrier, sealing these areas off from bacteria and food particles. Additionally, by filling in the deeper and more complex anatomy, sealants facilitate easier oral hygiene maintenance.

Sealants have been in clinical use for approximately three decades. The initial sealants were liquid resins applied to teeth and cured using ultraviolet light. However, modern sealants now use chemically-cured materials or alternative light sources for polymerization, which are safer and more efficient than ultraviolet light.

Most contemporary sealants are composed of Bowen's formula, known as BISGMA, which is a reaction product of bisphenol A and glycidyl methacrylate.[72] This material is also used in the matrix of composite resin filling materials.

Classification of sealants –

1. **Polymerization method:**
   A. Self - activation (mixing two components)
   B. Light-activation
      - First generation: ultraviolet light
      - Second generation: Dual cure
      - Third generation: visible light
      - Fourth generation: fluoride releasing.[72]

2. **Resin system**
   - BIS-GMA
   - Urethane acrylate

3. **Filled and Unfilled**

4. **Clear or tinted**

Requisites of an ideal sealant:

1. A viscosity allowing penetration into deep and narrow fissures even in the maxillary teeth.
2. Adequate working time.
3. Rapid cure.
4. Good and prolonged adhesion to enamel.
5. Low absorption and solubility.
6. Resistance to wear.
7. Minimum irritation to tissues.
8. Cariostatic action.

Indications

- Recently emerged permanent bicuspids and molars exhibiting complete recession of the pericoronal operculum, along with open or adhesive grooves and fissures.
- Discoloured pits and fissures showing minimal decalcification or cloudiness, with no softness detected at the base of fissures.
- Presence of caries or previous extraction of teeth due to caries in a child's dentition indicates an increased risk of caries, warranting consideration for sealant application.
- Similarly, if a young adult necessitates restoration of one second molar, sealing the remaining second molars appears to be a sensible preventive measure.
- A fissure pattern characterized by shallow, rounded grooves is less prone to decay, whereas deep fissures are more susceptible due to difficulties in cleaning.[72]

Contraindications

- Individuals with no history of caries and well-merged pit and fissure anatomy.
- Teeth showing radiographic or clinical signs of caries on the proximal surfaces should not undergo sealing.
- Wide pits and fissures that are self-cleansing.
- Teeth that are difficult to isolate or are partially erupted.
- Pits and fissures that have remained free of caries for four years or more.[72]

Advantages

- Esthetic value.
- Low thermal conductivity.
- No galvanic reactions.
- Placed in one appointment.
- Easily repaired.
- Bonded resin may enhance tooth strength.
- Conservative preparation technique minimizes loss of healthy tooth structure.
- Some materials release fluoride.

Disadvantages

- Lacks self-sealing ability, unlike amalgam.
- Leakage occurs with a high rate of secondary caries because of the breakage of the adhesive-tooth bond.
- Excessive wear under stress.
- Low fracture strength.
- High technique sensitivity.
- Generation and inhalation of dust during finishing procedures represent a potential hazard for patient and dental staff.
- Polymerization shrinkage of some composites may cause bacterial leakage and high stress to develop in the tooth.
- Increased plaque adhesion.
- Allergenic potential.

Sealant Application Technique[75]

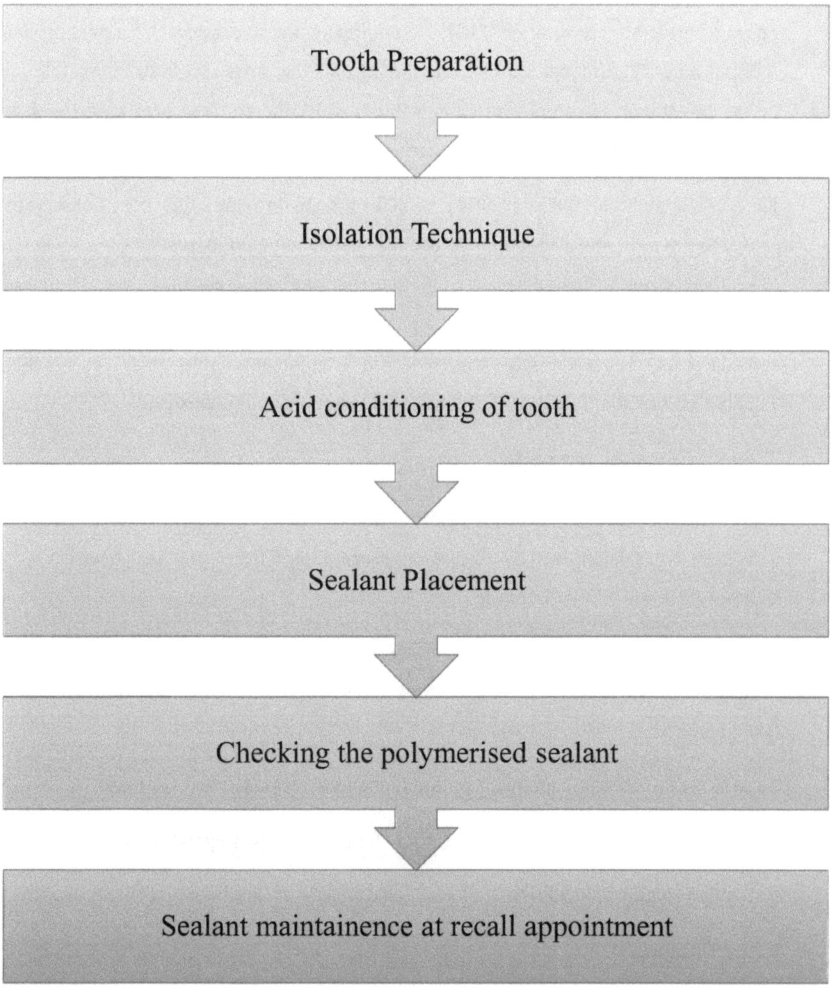

6.2 Preventive Resin Restoration

The preventive resin restoration (PRR) is a minimally invasive approach for treating small occlusal caries. This procedure entails removing only the carious tooth structure, followed by the placement of composite resin. Subsequently, the restored area along with the remaining unaffected pits and fissures are sealed using a fissure sealant.[13]

The development of the preventive resin technique provides the most conservative approach towards confined, incipient occlusal caries in young permanent teeth whereby restoration occurs with a minimum of tooth preparation while ensuring the prevention of future caries formation through sealant placement. The resin placed in the caries areas and adjacent caries susceptible areas seal them from the oral environment and provide a valuable treatment alternative to conventional restorations like amalgam.

Types of preventive resin restoration:

There are three types of preventive resin restorations based on the extent and depth of the carious lesion as determined by exploratory preparation. These types have been classified as types A, B ·and C by Simonsen.

Type A comprises suspicious pits and fissures where caries removal is limited to enamel. A slow-speed round bur is used to remove any decalcified enamel, and local anesthesia is not required.

Type B is defined as the incipient lesion in dentin that is small and confined.

Type C is characterized by the need for greater exploratory preparation of depth. This restoration requires the administration of local anesthetic and liner placement over the exposed dentin.

Initially, Simonsen advocated an unfilled sealant for type A, a diluted composite resin for type B, and a filled composite resin for type C. The concept of a diluted composite resin, which is a mixture of filled composite resin and an unfilled bonding agent has a superior retention due to the greater wear resistance of the filled resin particles, whereas the dilution with the unfilled resin provided the necessary viscosity for flow.

Technique:

Placement of preventive resin restoration utilizes principles of acid etch technique similar to those of sealant placement with the exception of caries removal from isolated pits and fissures. Higher retention rates are attributed to the fact that fissure enlargement results in increased surface layer for etching, elimination of the organic material surface layer and a thicker sealant.[1]

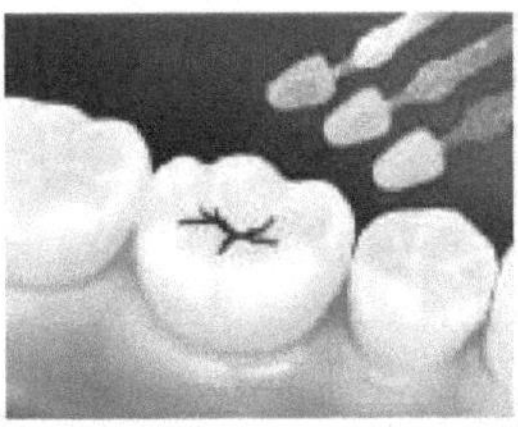

1. Shade selection

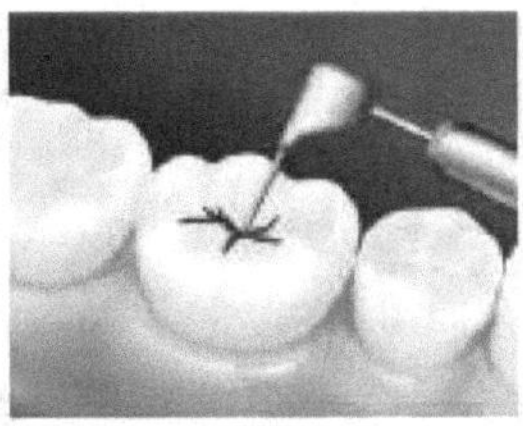

2. Preparation

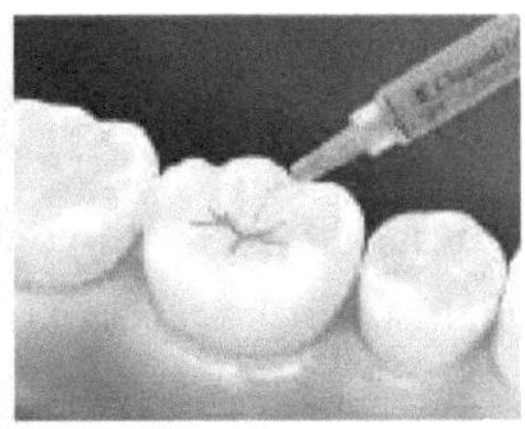

3. Etching

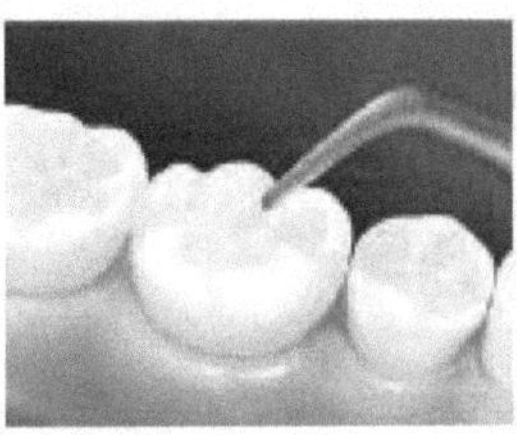

4. Cleaning and dry

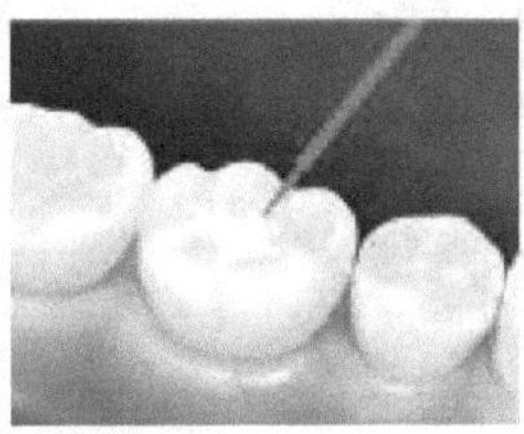

5. Bonding

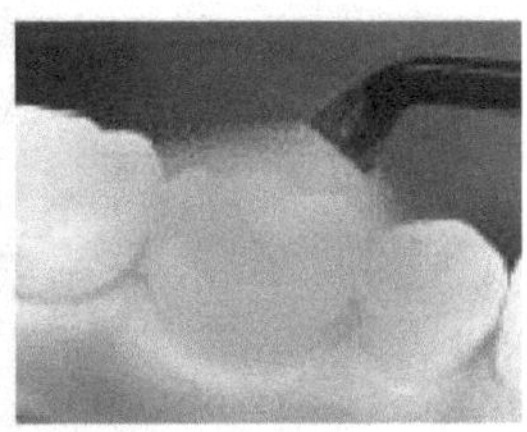

6. Light Curing (20sec)

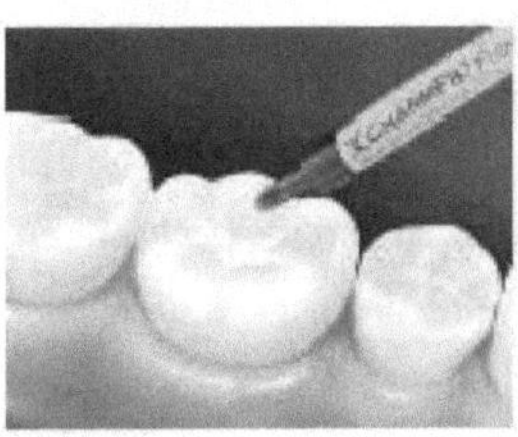

7. Filling

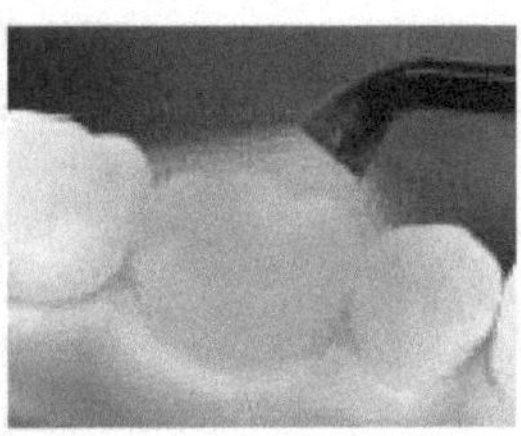

8. Light Curing

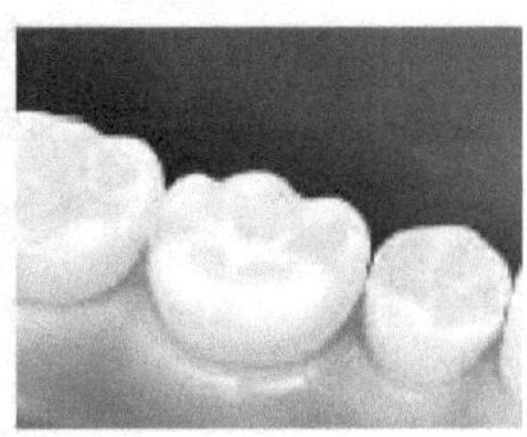

9. Polishing

Advantages of PRR

1. Minimal cavity preparation is required thus prevents unnecessary removal of healthy tooth structure for retention.
2. Seals caries thereby halting the destruction of tooth e.g. teeth with pits and fissures.
3. Risk of microleakage is reduced.
4. Loss of the restoration and subsequent replacement proves to be less invasive than that for conventional restoration like amalgam.

Precaution:

Early loss of preventive resin restoration similar to fissure sealant has been attributed to insufficient etching. Thus it is very important to maintain excellent isolation from salivary and moisture contamination for the long term success of Preventive Resin Restoration.[1]

Selectively invasive interventions :-

Extended fissure sealants

Pit & Fissure carious lesions in permanent molars account for over 80% of the total carious experience seen in children & adolescents. Teeth are especially at risk of developing caries in the fissures within the 1st 3 years after eruption as pits & fissures are havens for plaque retention & are impossible to clean when they have a narrow & deep morphology. Epidemiological studies showed that the sealing of pit & fissures is an effective approach to prevent pit & fissure caries. To achieve an optimal caries protective effect, the whole fissure system must be sealed completely without leaving any gaps.

A pit and fissure sealant is defined as a material that is introduced into the occlusal pits and fissures of caries-susceptible teeth, thus forming a micromechanically-bonded, protective layer, cutting access of caries-producing bacteria from their source of nutrients.

Robertson stated in 1835 that the caries potential was directly related to the shape and depth of the pits and fissures and caries seldom began on smooth, easily cleaned surfaces. Buonocore's classic study of 1955 marked the start of a major revolution in the clinical practice of dentistry. The first clinical benefit from Buonocore's work was the introduction of the first dental pit and fissure sealant, Nuva-seal (L.D. Caulk) in February 1971, along with its curing initiator and ultraviolet light source, the Caulk Nuva Lite.

Age ranges for extended sealant application:

A high percentage of occlusal lesions occurred in the first 3 years after eruption.

- 3-4 years of age for the primary molar sealant application
- 6-7 years of age for the permanent first molar
- 11-13 years of age for the permanent second molar

6.3 Miniature implants versus standard-size implants

A Mini Dental Implant (MDI), a titanium implant resembling a miniature tooth root, is notably slimmer than traditional implants. Initially devised for securing dentures, they gained recognition as permanent fixtures following FDA clearance in April 1999. Dentists increasingly favor MDIs for denture stabilization and as alternatives for crown support in limited space scenarios. They typically cost one-fourth to one-third of standard implants.[76]

Diverse jawbone physiologies necessitate varying implant platform widths. Narrower implants, such as MDIs, find utility in front areas, while wider ones are preferred for premolars and molars due to greater lateral forces. MDIs, available in diameters of 1.8mm to 2.9mm and various lengths, offer flexibility based on bone density and location.[77]

In the posterior region of the mouth, specifically the premolars and molars, where lateral forces exert the greatest pressure and tooth strength is paramount, dentists typically opt for wide platform dental implants ranging from 4.5mm to 6mm in diameter. Utilizing a wider platform enables the dentist to construct a robust, secure tooth supported by the dense and substantial bone capable of withstanding the considerable forces and stresses present in this area of the mouth.[76]

Mini implants are available in four diameters: 1.8mm, 2.1mm, 2.4mm, and 2.9mm, each diameter offered in four lengths: 10mm, 13mm, 15mm, and 18mm. The 2.9mm diameter mini implant is termed a "Hybrid" because it closely approximates the diameter of the smallest root form implant available, yet can still be placed using the simplified surgical technique outlined below. Hybrids are specifically designed for use in the softer bone densities typically found in the upper arch, while smaller diameter implants are more suited to denser bone types. Surgeons determine the implant length based on the vertical bone available to support it, with very dense cortical bone favouring shorter, thinner implants. Typically, four mini implants are positioned in the anterior section of the lower jaw.[76]

Unlike standard implants, mini implants permit immediate loading, enabling patients to leave the office on the day of surgery with a securely stable lower denture that can be used for eating immediately. Mini implants often allow for placement in the lower jaw without the need for incisions in the gums, as they can be inserted directly through the gums into the underlying bone. Anesthesia is generally required only at the specific gum locations where each implant is to be inserted.[76]

MDIs permit immediate loading, enabling patients to use stabilized dentures promptly post-surgery. Unlike traditional implants, MDIs often require no gum incisions and can be inserted directly into the bone, reducing procedure time and discomfort. Integration occurs swiftly, allowing immediate denture use without prolonged waiting periods.[77] The procedure, taking about 90 minutes, is minimally invasive with few contraindications. Patients benefit from immediate denture stability, facilitated by MDIs' immediate integration and minimal post-operative discomfort.[76]

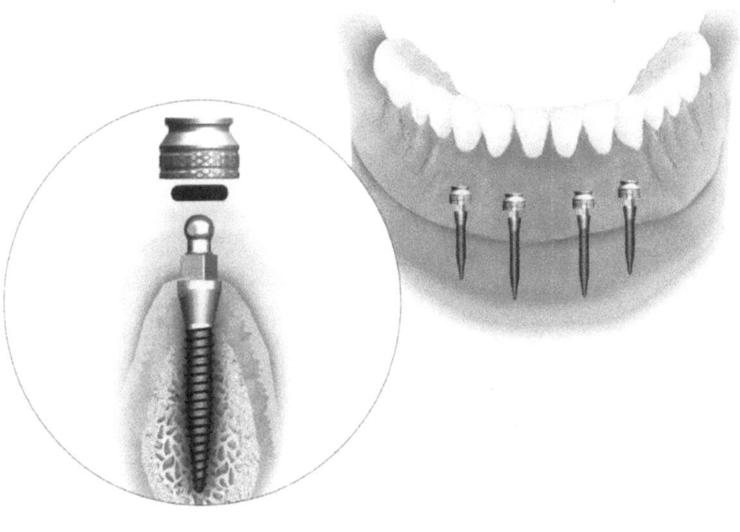

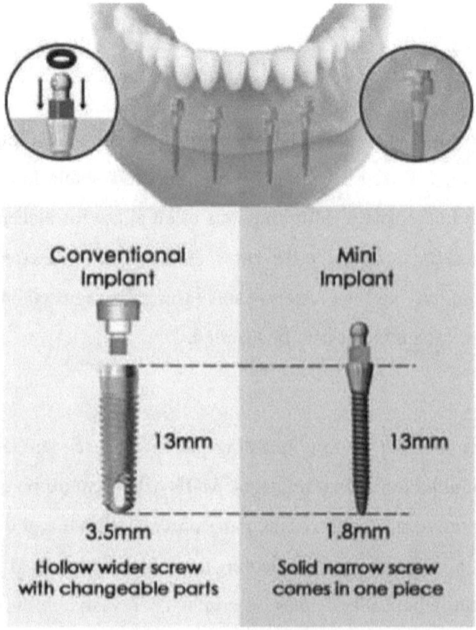

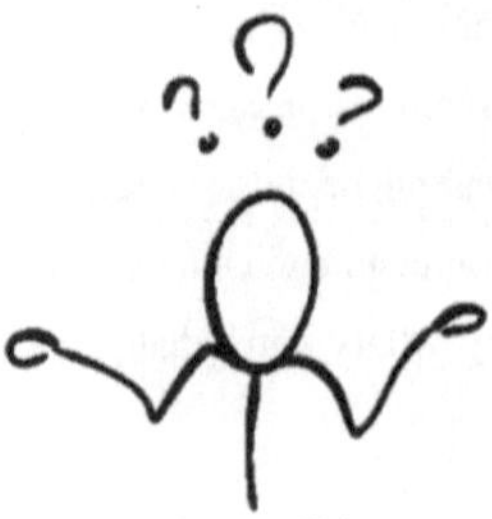

What is the typical lifespan of mini implants?

It's impossible to provide a precise guarantee for the longevity of any implant due to the multitude of patient-specific factors involved. Using the term "permanent" to describe medical or dental devices is inaccurate, as nothing in medicine or dentistry can be guaranteed to endure indefinitely. The term "long term" is more appropriate and truthful when discussing dental appliances. Some mini implants placed as far back as the mid-1970s are still functioning today. Mini implants became widely used around the year 2000 after FDA approval for long-term use.

The vast majority of MDI minis installed since then continue to function effectively. However, a small percentage of implants may fail for various reasons. Fortunately, removing a failed mini implant is straightforward, and healing typically occurs without complications. Another implant can usually be inserted immediately adjacent to the site of the failed implant or, if preferred, after a three-month waiting period directly into the former implant location.

6.4 Placement of inlays and onlays instead of crowns

Restorative dentistry stands as a distinct sector within cosmetic dentistry, concentrating on the repair and replacement of deteriorated or damaged teeth. Among the frequently employed techniques by cosmetic dentists to restore damaged teeth are the crafting and placement of tooth crowns and dental bridges. The transformative effects these treatments can have on damaged teeth are remarkable.[78] Inlays and onlays, for instance, offer enhanced strength and durability compared to traditional fillings while remaining more cost-effective than crowns.

What is a dental crown?

When a tooth sustains damage beyond the capacity for a filling, a dental crown may become necessary. A crown is a custom-made tooth-shaped covering that is placed over a damaged or decayed tooth.

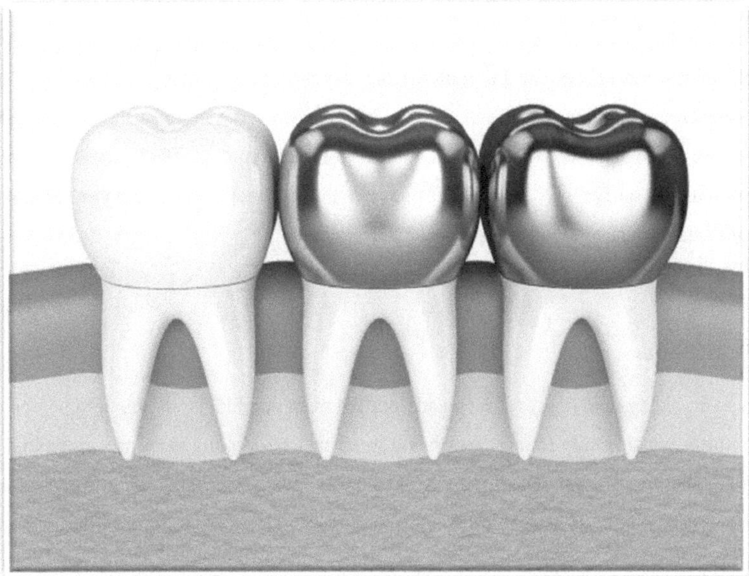

Inlays:

Inlays are utilized to address decay or damage present on the top surfaces of teeth. Typically, inlay placement involves two visits to your cosmetic dentist. During the initial visit, an impression of the affected tooth is taken, and a temporary inlay is fitted onto the tooth. The impression is then sent to a dental laboratory, where the permanent inlay is meticulously crafted to match the specifications of your tooth. Upon your return to the dentist, the temporary inlay is removed, and the permanent one is securely placed over the tooth.

Onlays:

Onlays are employed to treat decay that extends to one or more of the cusps (the top projections of the tooth). The process for onlay placement closely mirrors that of inlays, beginning with an impression being taken and a temporary onlay being affixed to the tooth during the initial visit. The impression is then sent to a dental lab, where a dental technician fabricates the onlay according to the tooth's dimensions. On the subsequent visit to the dentist, the temporary restoration is removed, and the permanent onlay is bonded securely to the tooth using high-strength dental resins.

Both inlays and onlays can be crafted from tooth-coloured materials, rendering them virtually imperceptible to the naked eye. They also preserve more of the natural tooth structure since their application necessitates minimal removal of the tooth's surface. Additionally, onlays can help patients avoid the eventual need for more extensive treatments such as crowns, bridges, or dental implants.

Advantages:

Given that inlays and onlays are typically crafted from durable, tooth-coloured porcelain, they offer considerably longer-lasting and more natural-looking outcomes compared to the metal fillings employed in the past. Dentists can securely bond them to the tooth's surface, enhancing structural integrity and preventing bacteria from infiltrating and forming cavities.

Advantages of inlays and onlays over metal fillings:

- They enhance the strength of the tooth they fill by forming a permanent bond with it, unlike metal fillings. Porcelain fillings reinforce the tooth structure by distributing forces across the bonded surfaces, while metal fillings exert outward pressure on the tooth's periphery due to their tightly packed placement within the cavity, gradually weakening the tooth and potentially leading to cracks.

- They are non-reactive to hot and cold substances in the mouth, unlike metal fillings. Metal amalgam fillings, comprising about half mercury along with other metals, exhibit thermal expansion and contraction upon exposure to hot and cold stimuli, thereby exerting repeated stress on the tooth and contributing to its gradual weakening over time.

- They offer permanent retention and do not risk loosening or falling out over time, a concern associated with aging metal fillings. Porcelain inlays and onlays form a seamless bond with the tooth and become an integral part of it, ensuring long-term stability.

- They provide an aesthetically pleasing appearance, as the porcelain used can be precisely matched to the natural shade of your teeth. Superior dental laboratories even employ multiple shades of porcelain within the same restoration to mimic the subtle variations in tooth enamel. Moreover, the porcelain, like natural enamel, exhibits light-reflecting properties, resulting in a youthful and healthy smile.

6.5 Chemo mechanical method of caries removal

Chemo mechanical removal of dental caries entails softening dental caries chemically using N-monochloro-DL-2-aminobutyric acid (NMAB) or N-monochloroglycine (NMG) at a pH range of 11.2-11.4, followed by the selective removal of carious material through gentle mechanical excavation. This method has been developed as a potential alternative to the traditional mechanical removal of carious dentine. The reagent is created by combining amino butyric acid or glycine with sodium hypochlorite, and its mechanism of action purportedly involves chlorination and disruption by NMAB or NMG of the partially degraded collagen fibres found in carious dentine. The application of NMAB or NMG to carious dentine softens the layer containing denatured collagen, making it more fragile and enabling its selective removal through gentle excavation.[24,79]

However, the current procedure has limitations concerning treatment duration, cavity suitability, and the continued necessity for some mechanical instrument use, necessitating selective application. More recently, two in vitro studies with well-controlled parameters have indicated that NMAB is no more effective than saline or water in removing carious dentine in permanent teeth. These findings raise doubts about the validity of prior clinical trials that did not account for factors such as applied force and criteria for caries removal assessment. Additionally, the commercial applicator system utilizing the CaridexTM unit was found to have inadequate thermostatic and flow rate control.[79]

Chemo mechanical Methodology:

The foundation of chemo mechanical caries removal traces back to the research conducted by Goldman and Kronman in New Jersey, United States. Initially introduced in 1972 as the Original GK-101 solution, the chemo-mechanical approach comprised a formula primarily composed of N-MonochloroGlycine (NMG) and sodium hypochlorite.

However, GK-101 proved to be insufficiently efficient in caries removal rate, leading to its evolution into GK-101E. In this iteration, glycine was substituted with amino butyric acid, resulting in the product N-monochloroaminobutyric acid (NMAB). The NMAB system was patented in the US in 1975, with further patents obtained by the National Patent Dental Corporation in New York in 1987.[80] It received FDA approval for use in the USA in 1984 and was commercialized as CaridexTM. This system comprised two solutions: solution I containing sodium hypochlorite and solution II containing glycine, amino butyric acid, sodium chloride, and sodium hydroxide. The two solutions were mixed immediately before use to form the working reagent (pH approximately 11), which remained stable for one hour.

This caries removal system encompassed a solution (GK-101E), reservoir, heater, pump, handpiece, and an applicator tip affixed to the handpiece.[81]

The Caridex system had certain clinical limitations, including efficacy of caries removal, the substantial volume of solution required, short shelf life, and the duration of the procedure. To address these shortcomings, Medi Team in Sweden developed a new method for chemo mechanical caries removal in January 1998, branded as CaisolvTM.[82] Marketed in two syringes, one containing sodium hypochlorite solution and the other a pink viscous gel comprising three amino acids (lysine, leucine, and glutamic acid), along with carboxymethyl-cellulose to increase viscosity and erythrosine to enhance visibility during use. The contents of the two syringes are mixed using a simple system, joining them immediately before use, as effectiveness begins to diminish after 20 minutes.[81]

	Caridex	**Carisolv**
Solution – I	1% NaOCl	0.5% NaOCl
Solution – II	0.1 M aminobutyric acid glycine 0.1 M NaCl 0.1 M NaOH	0.1 M glutamic acid / leucine / lysine NaCl NaOH
Dye	-	Erythrocin(pink)
pH	11	11
Physical properties	Liquid	Gel
Volume needed	100-500 ml	0.2 - 1.0 ml
Time required	5-15 minutes	5-15 minutes
Equipment required	Applicator unit	None
Instruments	Applicator tips	Specially designed
Preparation remains active after mixing	1 hour	20 minutes

Advantages of Chemo mechanical Caries Removal System:

1. This method circumvents the painful removal of healthy dentin while remaining ineffective in eliminating hard eburnated portions of the lesion; however, the removal of eburnated caries may not be imperative.

2. There is a diminished requirement for anesthesia, with preservation of intact tooth structure and a reduced likelihood of pulp exposure. It is particularly suitable for treating apprehensive patients, those with medical conditions, and paediatric dentistry.

3. The instrument utilized in chemo mechanical caries removal reduces the risk of inadvertently removing intact dentin compared to conventional excavators or drills.

4. The dentinal surface treated via chemo mechanical means is ideally compatible with adhesive restorative materials, potentially eliminating the need for acid etching.

5. The application of this technique, devoid of reliance on electricity or expensive dental equipment, enables cost-effective treatment for larger populations.

Disadvantages of Chemo mechanical Caries Removal System:

1. Some patients find the taste of the solution unpleasant.
2. Rotary instruments may still be necessary for removing tissue or materials other than degraded dentin collagen.
3. The time required for complete caries removal is prolonged.
4. Rotary instruments are indispensable for accessing carious dentin to facilitate the function of the gel.
5. The surface energy of chemo mechanically treated dentin is elevated, attracting contaminants, which may necessitate the use of a rubber dam.

6.6 Atraumatic Restorative Treatment(ART)

The Atraumatic Restorative Treatment (ART) is a technique centred around the manual removal of carious cavities within teeth using solely hand instruments, followed by the restoration of these cavities using an adhesive filling material, typically glass ionomer.

Hand Instruments Utilized in ART :-

ART is employed in scenarios where traditional restorative treatments are impractical. Its aim is to halt the progression of tooth decay until more definitive care can be provided or until the need for treatment ceases due to natural tooth shedding. By removing decayed tooth structure and promoting remineralization of affected dentin (without infection), ART effectively reduces bacterial load. It equips oral health practitioners with a means to uphold the principle of "Teeth for Life."[67]

The use of hand instruments alone for caries removal and subsequent restoration with glass ionomer allows for maximal preservation of tooth structure and prevents further decay. ART employs straightforward yet efficient techniques involving manual instrumentation and slow-speed rotary preparation.[67] It relies on materials with low sensitivity to technique, particularly crucial for treating young children with limited attention spans. The procedure is typically swift and does not necessitate local anesthesia, making it advantageous for paediatric cases.

In instances where behavioral challenges or other factors preclude the use of conventional restorative dentistry (such as cost constraints or parental preferences against pharmacological interventions), ART may serve as a viable treatment option. However, it is important to acknowledge that ART does have its limitations.

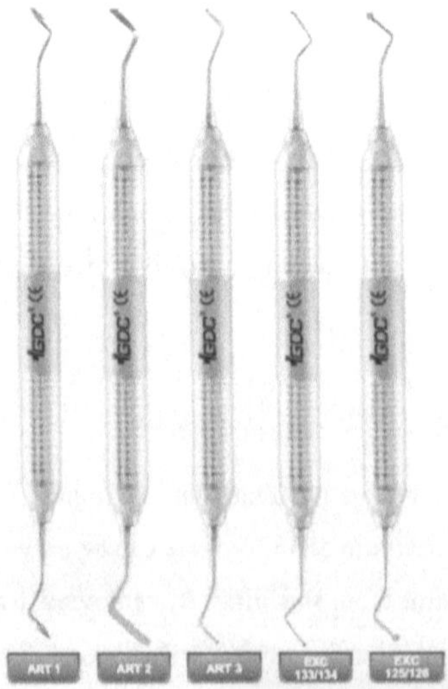
ART 1
ART 2
ART 3
EXC 133/134
EXC 125/128

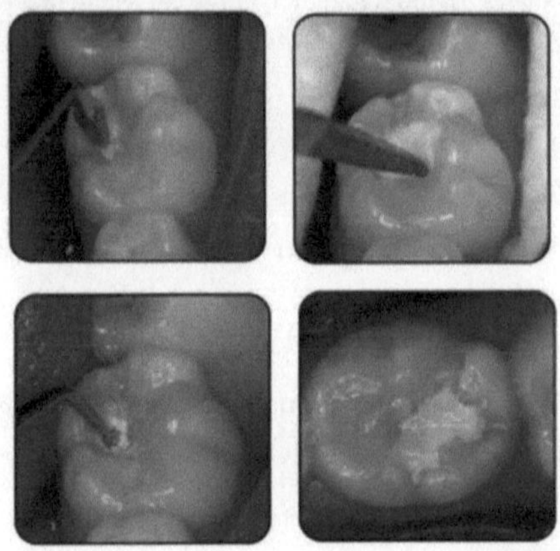

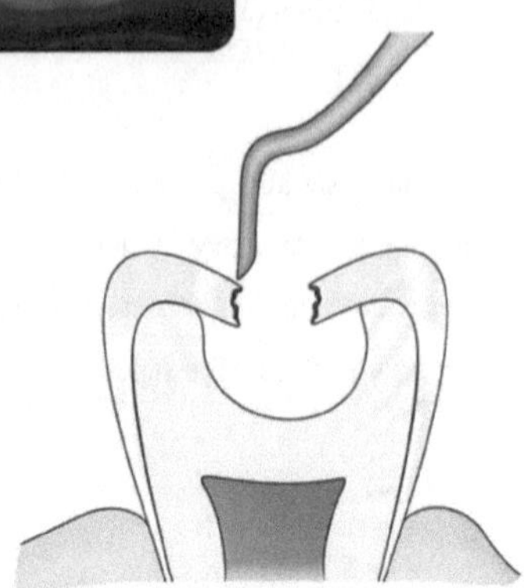

The fundamental principles of ART encompass:

- Utilizing hand instruments exclusively for the removal of carious tooth tissue
- Restoring the cavity with glass ionomer material.

The rationale behind employing hand instruments instead of electrically driven handpieces includes:

- Ensuring accessibility of restorative care to diverse population groups.
- Adopting a biological approach that involves minimal cavity preparation, thus preserving healthy tooth structures and minimizing tooth trauma.
- Cost-effectiveness of hand instruments in comparison to electrically driven dental equipment.
- Minimizing pain, thereby reducing the necessity for local anesthesia and mitigating psychological distress in patients.
- Streamlined infection control procedures, as hand instruments can be readily cleaned and sterilized after each patient encounter.[67]

Reasons for using glass ionomers include Restoration longevity, Moisture tolerance, Esthetic properties.[83]

Regarding factors influencing ART failures:

1. **Material factors** encompass issues related to the composition, quality, and properties of the materials used in the restoration process, including inadequate adhesion, insufficient strength, or premature wear.
2. **Operator factors** involve skill level, experience, and adherence to proper technique during the ART procedure, which can impact the success of the restoration.
3. **Technique factors** refer to aspects of the treatment approach, such as inadequate cavity preparation, improper placement of the restoration, or insufficient isolation, which may contribute to suboptimal outcomes.

ART Failure	**Management**
Partial Material Loss	Cleaning fracture surface, Application of dentine conditioner, Placement of new GIC Layer.
Complete Material Loss	Cleaning cavity surface, Application of dentine conditioner, Placement of new GIC Layer.
Caries related to restoration margin	Caries removal using hand excavator, Cleaning GIC surface, Application of dentine conditioner, Placement of new GIC Layer.

Advantages:

1. Soft, demineralized dentin and friable enamel are selectively removed without the use of rotary instruments, resulting in minimal cavity preparation and conservation of tooth tissue.
2. Both pits and fissures, along with the cavity itself, can be filled or sealed using the restorative material.
3. The procedure typically involves little to no pain, reducing the need for local anesthesia.
4. Anxiety commonly associated with traditional restorative procedures is minimized.
5. Only inexpensive and readily available hand instruments are utilized, simplifying infection control measures.
6. The overall cost of the procedure is relatively low.

Limitations:

1. Long-term survival rates for glass ionomer ART restorations and sealants have not been extensively studied; the longest reported study duration is three years. Acceptance of the technique among oral health care professionals is not guaranteed.
2. Currently, the technique is limited to treating small to medium-sized, one-surface lesions due to the lower wear resistance and strength of existing glass ionomer materials.
3. Prolonged use of hand instruments may lead to hand fatigue.
4. Hand mixing may result in variations in the consistency of the glass ionomer mix among operators and in different geographical or climatic conditions.
5. There is a misconception that ART is an easily performed procedure; in reality, each step must be executed meticulously.
6. The perceived simplicity of the technique may hinder its acceptance within the dental profession.
7. Some members of the public may mistakenly view the new glass ionomer "white fillings" as temporary dressings.

6.7 Digital radiography versus conventional radiography

Digital radiography involves using digital X-ray sensors instead of traditional photographic film for imaging purposes. This approach offers several advantages, including enhanced time efficiency by eliminating the need for chemical processing and the capability to digitally transfer and improve images. Additionally, digital radiography allows for the use of lower radiation levels while maintaining similar contrast to conventional radiography.

Electronic imaging technology has been accessible for over a decade, with the pioneering direct digital imaging system, RadioVisioGraphy (RVG), developed by Dr. Frances Mouyens and produced by Trophy Radiology in 1984.[84] It was introduced in the U.S. dental literature in 1989. Digital imaging relies on X-ray interactions with electrons in electronic sensor pixels, conversion of analogue data to digital format, computer processing, and the display of the resulting image on a computer screen.

Data collected by the sensor is transmitted to the computer in analogue form. Computers operate using the binary number system, employing two digits (0 and 1) known as bits to represent data. These bits form words, which are typically eight bits or more in length and are called bytes.[85]

Direct digital imaging systems generate dynamic images that allow for immediate display, enhancement, storage, retrieval, and transmission of images.

Advantages and Disadvantages :-

Charge coupled devices (CCDs) offer several advantages over traditional film, including reduced exposure, elimination of processing chemicals, instantaneous image production and display, enhanced image quality, patient education benefits, and convenient storage. The extent of exposure reduction depends on various factors such as film speed, sensor size, collimation, and the need for retakes.

However, CCDs also come with some drawbacks. These include the rigidity and thickness of the sensor, decreased resolution, higher initial system cost, uncertainty regarding sensor lifespan, and the challenge of perfect semiconductor charge transfer. Infection control poses another challenge, as CCD sensors cannot be sterilized. Proper preparation, coverage, and barrier protection during patient imaging procedures are essential to prevent damage.

Diagnostic Utility of Digital Imaging

Several studies have explored the effectiveness of digital imaging compared to film-based imaging in diagnosing various dental conditions, including caries, periodontal disease, and periapical lesions. Overall, these studies consistently show that film and digital imaging modalities do not significantly differ in their ability to detect dental diseases.

In 1998, Wenzel conducted a review of the evidence on the diagnostic efficacy of digital imaging systems for caries detection.[85] The conclusion drawn was that digital imaging systems appear to be equally accurate as film for diagnosing caries in general.

Indirect or Scanned Digital Imaging

Direct digital imaging involves capturing the original image in a digital format, where the image consists of discrete units of information known as pixels.

Indirect photostimulable phosphor plates (PSP) imaging is another form of digital imaging. With PSP, the image is initially captured on a phosphor plate as analogue information, which is then converted into a digital format during processing. Several studies have assessed the diagnostic usefulness of PSP systems, with most reporting comparable results between PSP and conventional film images. For instance, Svanaes et al. found no difference in proximal caries detection between PSP and Ektaspeed film, while Cederberg et al. concluded that PSP images outperformed conventional Ektaspeed film images in determining endodontic working lengths.[86,87] One significant advantage of PSP image receptors is their cordless nature, which greatly facilitates their placement.

Extraoral Imaging

Extraoral digital imaging can be achieved using either direct or indirect digital imaging systems. Various panoramic systems are available, utilizing linear array CCD or PSP plate sensors. When considering a digital panoramic system, factors such as sensor cost, image capture time, and file size need to be taken into account.

Digital Subtraction Radiography

In the realm of dentistry, Digital subtraction radiography emerges as a solution, enabling the precise quantification of changes in radiographic images.[84] The principle behind digital subtraction radiography is relatively straightforward. Initially, a radiographic image is captured before a specific treatment is administered. Subsequently, another image is obtained after the treatment. Both images are digitized and meticulously compared on a pixel-by-pixel basis. The resulting image showcases only the alterations that have occurred, effectively "subtracting" unchanged components from the visual representation. One of the primary benefits afforded by direct digital imaging (including PSP) is the consistency of image file sizes across the board.

DICOM Standard

DICOM, which stands for Digital Imaging and Communications in Medicine, is currently at version 3.0. This standardization aims to facilitate the transfer of digital information to both remote locations and local workstations by establishing standardized formats. While dentistry is gradually acknowledging the DICOM 3.0 standard, its uniform implementation remains inconsistent. This becomes especially critical when considering digital image submissions to insurance providers or ensuring compatibility among various office software systems, such as dental records and voice-activated charting.[88]

Several studies have highlighted numerous advantages of direct digital radiography over conventional film radiography:

1. Dynamic Image Adjustments: Unlike film, digital images offer dynamic adjustments in contrast and density tailored to the diagnostic task, potentially reducing the need for retakes.

2. Enhanced Dynamic Range: Direct digital receptors, particularly phosphor plates, possess a broader dynamic range compared to film, potentially minimizing retakes.

3. Elimination of Wet Processing: Direct digital systems eliminate the need for wet processing with chemical solutions, leading to fewer retakes and reduced environmental impact. Additionally, this eliminates the costs associated with film and chemicals.

4. Reduced Radiation Dose: Direct digital systems typically require 5 to 50% less radiation dose than conventional radiography to achieve acceptable image quality. Consequently, population doses from dental diagnostics can be significantly reduced, prolonging the lifespan of X-ray tubes.

5. Accelerated Workflow: Direct digital systems significantly reduce the time from image exposure to display.

6.8 Cavity designs for minimal intervention

A. Fissurotomy

Managing fissures in posterior teeth has long posed a challenge for dentists due to the dilemma surrounding cavity preparation techniques. The fissurotomy bur presents a novel approach to ultra-conservative dental treatment. Specifically designed in shape and size, this bur is intended for treating superficial pits and fissure lesions while preserving the natural integrity of tooth structure by minimizing unnecessary loss of enamel and dentin.[29] This tapered bur features a head length of 2.5mm, allowing for the preparation of conservative cavities. Additionally, the fissurotomy kit (S.S. White, Lakewood NJ) includes acid etchant (37% orthophosphoric acid), bonding agent (Excite), and a flowable composite (Helimolar) capable of efficiently flowing into all crevices and fissures.[29]

Unlike traditional cutting burs, which remove a significant amount of enamel regardless of the depth of the cut and are aimed at accessing caries that has advanced beyond the enamel-dentin junction (DEJ), the fissurotomy system adopts a notably more conservative approach.

Procedure

1) All pit and fissure areas are examined with a probe. Even if no obvious decay is detected, the fissures may exhibit a slightly tacky sensation upon exploration.

2) The specially designed fissurotomy bur is utilized to perform an incisional biopsy of all areas suspected of caries and those presenting with suspicious fissures.

3) Fissures are carefully examined for decay using the bur, while the surrounding enamel is contoured to create a gentle taper.

4) The tapered preparation is carried out, stopping just within the dentinoenamel junction (DEJ). If caries are shallow, it may not be necessary to reach the DEJ.

5) The restoration produced using this ultra-conservative method typically measures 1/8 to 1/10 of the intercuspal distance, in contrast to conventional amalgam restorations, which are about 1/3 of the intercuspal distance.

6) If there is any suspicion of residual caries, caries-detecting dye is applied and then rinsed off after 10 seconds. Any dentin stained red is subsequently removed.

7) A typical fissurotomy preparation exhibits a narrow, elongated, and irregularly deep configuration.

8) Finally, the prepared cavity is restored using flowable composites.[29]

Advantages:

A. The compact head length provides precise control for the dentist, ensuring that the bur tip cuts just beneath the DEJ without exceeding it.
B. The tapered design of the bur reduces contact with dentinal tubules, minimizing heat generation and vibration during cutting.
C. By limiting the use of the fissurotomy bur to enamel, patient discomfort is minimized, and the necessity for local anesthesia is eliminated.

B. Enamel Cavity

Since the inception of operative dentistry, it has been a foundational principle that a retention form should be established in the dentin layer. This was necessary because traditional restorative materials relied on mechanical retention provided by the forms cut into the resilient dentin.[22] When G.V. Black introduced the concept of box-form preparation, dental cutting instruments were not as advanced, requiring the removal of the underlying dentin layer to access the hard and brittle enamel within the fissures.

However, with the introduction of air turbines and carbide burs, it became feasible to prepare a box-form cavity solely within the enamel.

Principle

Enamel rods converge at their apical ends, forming a centripetal arrangement, while being supported at their bases by dentin. Consequently, when amalgam is placed in a cavity confined to the enamel layer, the restoration is indirectly supported by the surrounding dentin, alleviating concerns about the brittleness of enamel.[22]

Equipment

The procedure utilizes the smallest flat-end fissure bur made of tungsten carbide (No. 56) in a high-speed turbine handpiece.

For creating undercuts, the smallest inverted cone steel bur (No. 33½ or 3/0), mounted on a low-speed engine, is employed.

Technique:

1) Caries detection dye is applied to precisely locate sites affected by caries.
2) Carbide bur is used to cut all fissures associated with caries, ensuring the cavity width remains minimal.
3) Subsequently, slight undercuts are created on the bottom sidewalls using an inverted cone bur at points where enamel rods are most inclined inward, typically observed on the buccal and lingual branches of the fissure.
4) The shape of the enamel cavity is determined by the distribution of fissures connected to caries. If the fissures are continuous, the cavity is extended to cover the entire occlusal surface and sometimes even the buccal and lingual surfaces, if necessary. However, if the fissures are discontinuous, small, separate cavities are prepared for each decay of small sizes.
5) The prepared cavity is filled with silver amalgam using a filling instrument with a diameter of 0.7mm. A universal plugger, featuring an iron shaft that vibrates longitudinally due to alternating electric current, is utilized. Combination points, which have tips of two shapes (bud and rod) combined in one end, are employed.
6) The mixed amalgam, carried on the top of the prepared cavity, is packed using the slant of the vibrating bud, driven into the deep corners with the rod, and then compressed again with the bud for condensation, shaping, and burnishing.

Advantages:

- Cavity preparation without pain.
- Minimal loss of tooth surface, preserving tooth strength.
- Reduced risk of restoration loosening or leakage, as enamel is harder, less flexible, and more chemically resistant than dentin.
- Lower likelihood of marginal restoration fracture due to the small cavity width.
- Reduced time and labor required.
- More cost-effective.

C. Tunnel and Slot Preparations

Tunnel and slot preparations offer conservative approaches particularly suited for older patients. Slot preparations are recommended for lesions located within 2.5 mm of the marginal ridge.[89] Various materials such as glass ionomer, composite, or amalgam can be employed, with slot amalgams proving equally successful compared to traditional Class II amalgams. Additionally, if necessary, a preventive resin or glass ionomer restoration can be applied over the occlusal surface. In select cases where the lesion exceeds 2.5 mm from the marginal ridge, a tunnel preparation may be considered. Detailed instructions for this technique are available elsewhere.

Typically, initial access is gained through the fossa just medial to the marginal ridge, ensuring it is not under occlusal load. A small tapered cylinder bur is directed towards the lesion, followed by a long-shanked bur positioned more uprightly to improve visibility. Completion of the preparation involves the use of small round burs and hand instruments. Glass ionomer is preferred due to the likelihood of some demineralized interproximal areas remaining and the inability to bevel interproximal enamel.

In recent years, there has been a shift towards conservative cavity designs in restorative dentistry. The tunnel preparation, also known as internal oblique preparation, internal fossa preparation, internal occlusal diagonal, or internal preparation, aligns with this trend. Initially described in 1963 for restoring distal approximal surfaces of deciduous second molars, this technique aimed to preserve marginal ridge integrity and suggested the use of fluoride leachable silicate cement for its potential anticariogenic effects.[89]

In the 1980s, Hunt and Knight reintroduced the preparation as a more conservative alternative to conventional Class II cavity for treating primary proximal caries in posterior teeth.

Principle:

The principle behind tunnel restoration is to maintain the integrity of the marginal ridge during posterior proximal restorations.[80]

When caries is confined solely to the proximal side without affecting the occlusal surface, conventional access is typically gained through the occlusal surface. However, this approach involves creating an occlusal dovetail and compromising the integrity of the marginal ridge while preparing the proximal box. Such conventional restorations often result in excessive tooth loss and pose a risk to the structural integrity of the marginal ridges.

In tunnel preparations, access is achieved through the occlusal surface without compromising the marginal ridge.

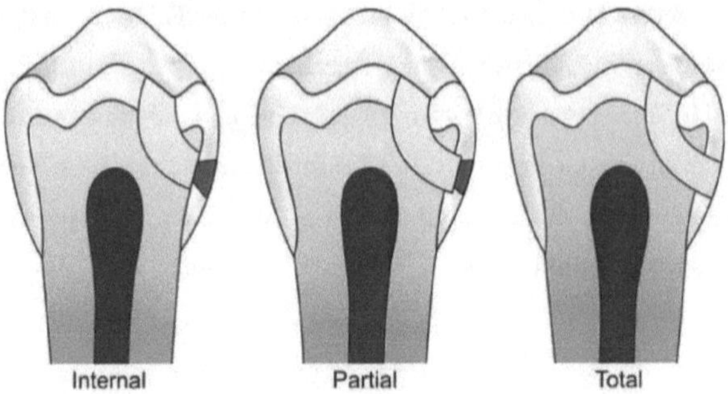

Technique:

1) Access is initiated through the mesial or distal pit, depending on the affected side.
2) Before cavity preparation, adjacent teeth are shielded using matrix bands.
3) For enhanced visual access, an orthodontic elastic separator is employed.
4) Starting from the relevant pit, approximately 2mm away from the marginal ridge, a small round bur is inserted through the pit, angling the bur at 45 degrees toward the proximal contact area.
5) As the lesion is approached, tapered fissure burs may be used to slightly widen the access.
6) The carious lesion is meticulously excavated by manoeuvring the bur in occlusal and gingival directions.
7) Throughout cavity preparation and restoration, the band is kept stable to prevent injury to adjacent teeth and underlying gingival tissue.
8) Subsequently, the prepared cavity is filled with a restorative material, typically glass ionomer cement (GIC), and if subjected to heavy occlusal forces, the 1mm occlusal segment is filled with composite resin.

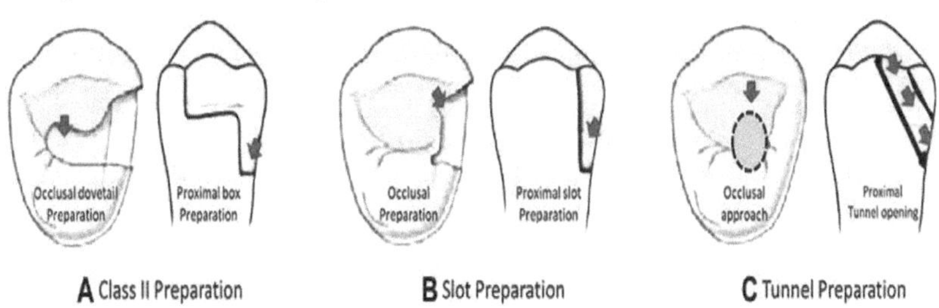

Advantages:

- Preservation of marginal ridge integrity, thereby upholding tooth strength.
- Preservation of a normal contact area is typically maintained.
- Minimal risk of overhang occurrence.
- Achieves an aesthetically pleasing outcome.
- Minimization of iatrogenic damage to adjacent teeth during preparation.
- Provision of fluoride supply to neighbouring tooth tissue.
- Reduced restorative perimeter resulting in decreased microleakage.
- Minimal impact on plaque accumulation and gingival/periodontal health.
- Cost-effectiveness.
- Potential for easy conversion to a conventional class preparation, if required.

Disadvantages:

- Achieving complete caries excavation may not be feasible.
- Potential for marginal ridge fracture exists.
- Restoration's marginal adaptability may be suboptimal.
- Higher likelihood of leakage and secondary caries.
- Insertion and finishing of the restorative material may pose challenges.
- Increased risk of secondary caries, especially in patients with high caries activity.

D. <u>Mini Box or Slot-Type Preparation</u>

The slot preparation, as proposed by Wilson and McLean, involves the elimination of the marginal ridge but excludes the occlusal pits and fissures if caries removal in these areas results in a box or saucer shape. Such preparations may be restored using Composite resin, Silver Amalgam, or Glass Ionomer Cement (GIC).[80] The facial slot Class II cavity preparation, initially introduced by Roggen Kamp and later adapted for GIC use by Crore, presents a time-saving, tooth-preserving, minimally invasive technique. It delivers an aesthetically pleasing restoration that is well-received by patients.

Principle

When a proximal lesion is near the marginal ridge, the entry to the carious lesion is established through the outer slope of the marginal ridge using a fine tapered fissure, preserving as much of the marginal ridge as feasible while minimizing disturbance to the contacts. Alternatively, a slot-type preparation with facial or lingual access has been recommended. However, when the carious lesion affects the interproximal contact area or requires extensive removal of sound tooth structure for access, occlusal access is preferred.

Technique

1) A Slot-type preparation with occlusal access entails entering the carious lesion and extending it gingivally, facially, and lingually.

2) Occlusal fissures are omitted from the preparation if they are caries-free.

3) For slot preparations intended for amalgam filling, ensuring definite undercut retention is crucial, although it is less critical when using composite resins.

4) A more conservative alternative is the 'Facial slot preparation' suitable for Class II lesions showing surface cavitation with radiographic evidence of caries extending 0.5mm into dentin.

5) Additionally, a minimum of 2mm of intact enamel must be present occluso-gingivally beneath the intact marginal ridge for facial slot preparation.

6) Proper isolation must be maintained to prevent contamination.

7) An interdental wedge is inserted just below the lesion. Access to the lesion is achieved using a slow-speed handpiece with a small-diameter round bur, following the DEJ occlusally, gingivally, and lingually using tactile skills.

8) If caries persist pulpally, a no. 329 bur is employed to remove softened dentin until space allows insertion of a small spoon excavator.

9) Lesion excavation continues until the spoon contacts dentin.

10) After cavity preparation, acid etching, bonding, and filling with composite resin or GIC are performed.

11) The Tofflemire matrix is loosely held in place until the restorative material is slightly overfilled using a nozzle. It is then tightened and left in position until the material sets.

12) Subsequently, the matrix is removed, and excess material is eliminated.

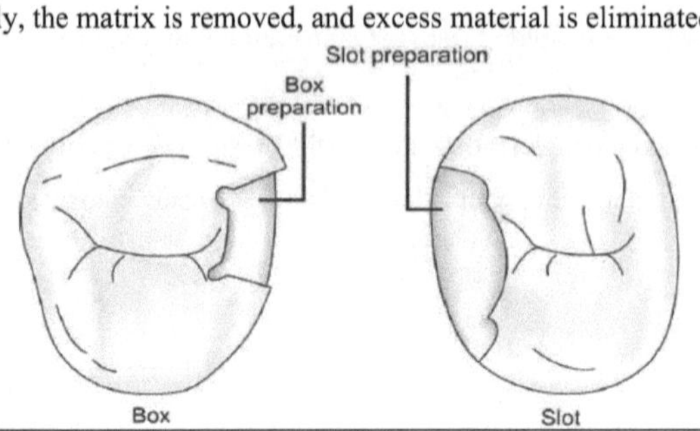

6.9 Lasers

Lasers stand as one of the most captivating advancements in medical technology. Within just a single generation, they have transitioned from the realm of imagination to becoming an integral part of everyday life. While lasers are not novel in dentistry, their exploration dates back to the 1960s, and today, a wide array of dental lasers and treatments are readily available.[90]

In contrast to ordinary light, where photons disperse in various wavelengths and directions, lasers possess distinctive qualities. They are monochromatic, coherent, and collimated. Laser light consists of a solitary wavelength, with its light waves synchronized and concentrated in a precise beam, rather than scattering in space.[50,52,90] These characteristics enable the concentration of an immense amount of energy into a small area. Hard tissue lasers, operating within the infrared range of the electromagnetic spectrum, are capable of cutting enamel, dentin, decay, and soft tissue.

Principle

When light interacts with matter, it can either be deflected or absorbed. If a photon is absorbed, its energy is not lost but rather utilized to elevate the energy level of the absorbing atom or molecule. Upon absorption, an electron within the atom or molecule transitions to a higher energy state, rendering the atom or molecule temporarily unstable. This state is referred to as an excited state, and the atom or molecule will eventually return to its ground state, releasing the stored energy in a process known as spontaneous emission.[90]

Lasing occurs when an excited atom is prompted to emit a photon before spontaneous emission takes place. When a photon with precisely the right energy interacts with an excited atom, it triggers the transition of the excited electron to a lower energy state, accompanied by the release of stored energy in the form of a second photon. This process, known as stimulated emission, results in two photons of identical wavelength traveling in the same direction.

If a greater number of atoms are pumped into an excited state than those remaining in the excited state, a population inversion occurs, which is a prerequisite for lasing. Consequently, within a confined space and at the speed of light, this photon chain reaction generates a brief but intense burst of monochromatic and coherent light.

In hydrokinetic laser systems, hydrokinetic energy is generated by combining a spray of atomized water with laser energy. Photons interact with water droplets surrounding the tip, causing them to fracture. The resulting energy allows for the gentle and precise removal of a wide range of human tissues, including tooth enamel.

Tools, Technique, and Procedure

Tools & Technique-

Currently, two manufacturers offer variations of Erbium lasers for cutting hard tissue. Biolase's Millennium features an Erbium, Chromium, Yttrium, Scandium, Gallium, and Garnet (Er, Cr: YSGG) laser with a wavelength of 2780nm. It operates by atomizing water droplets as they approach the target tissue. Laser energy induces micro-explosions in the water droplets, effectively separating and mechanically removing the surface target material in a gentle and atraumatic manner. This laser is equipped with a rotary handpiece design to access different areas of the mouth and maintains a fixed pulse repetition rate of 20Hz.[91]

Continuum Biomedical's De Light Dental Laser combines Erbium with Yttrium, Aluminium, and Garnet (Er: YAG) and operates at a wavelength of 2940nm. The DE Light emits pulses of light energy to micro-vaporize water within various target tissues, offering five preset power levels. Its thinner handpiece facilitates easier access and visualization of the work area. Additionally, the laser's frequency can be adjusted between 3Hz and 30Hz to enhance patient comfort according to the procedure. Its long, flexible delivery fibre ensures minimal resistance or drag, facilitating ease of use. Both lasers are employed for conservative preparations, aiding in the preservation of the tooth's structural integrity. They produce a tolerable, light popping noise during operation.

Procedure :

Different laser parameters or settings are necessary for ablating enamel, dentin, and caries due to the varying water content, which increases in enamel, dentin, and caries respectively. The Er wavelength, having an affinity for the water content of hard tissue, demands less energy to ablate caries compared to enamel or dentin due to its higher hydration.

When performing interproximal preparation, adjacent teeth should be isolated and protected using either a rubber dam or metal matrix.

↓

Utilize the smallest diameter tip that efficiently accomplishes the task.

↓

Gently touch the target tissue with the tip end, ensuring that cutting radiation emanates only from the distal end of the tip.

↓

Direct the water air stream onto the cutting tip and the target tissue.

↓

Always use the lowest possible power setting that achieves the goal in a timely manner.

↓

Maintain a wet operation area at all times.

↓

Mold the tip end to ensure efficient ablation and better tissue cooling.

↓

For wide cutting, continuously move the tip over the surface.

↓

Adjust the operating parameters during cavity preparation. For instance, when transitioning from ablating enamel to dentin, reposition the cutting tip 1mm from the tooth surface to decrease energy density and achieve slower ablation.

↓

If the patient becomes uncomfortable during the procedure, decrease pulses per second, energy, or switch the cutting tip from contact mode to non-contact mode.

↓

Employ an up-and-down pumping action for deep cutting.

↓

The laser system provides auditory feedback to the operator through characteristic 'popping' sounds, indicative of ablation.

↓

Laser cavity preparation typically results in an irregular shape, suitable for GIC or composite resin placement. However, line angles and point angles can be incorporated for enhanced mechanical retention.

An alternative laser usage technique proposed by Dr. Stewart P. Rosenberg suggests that the fastest and most efficient cutting occurs when the laser tip is positioned 1 to 1.5mm from the target tissue surface, known as the 'active cutting zone'. Deviating from this range diminishes the cutting effectiveness. Moving closer than 1 to 1.5mm may muffle the hydrokinetic effect, reducing cutting efficiency and potentially causing discomfort due to the transfer of raw laser energy without adequate hydrokinetic association with the water spray.

Advantages of Lasers in Restorative Dentistry:

- Lasers enhance the restorative process by making it more conservative and precise.
- Patients experience less trauma during the procedure, resulting in reduced operative time.
- Anesthesia is often unnecessary, eliminating discomfort associated with numb lips or tongue.
- Multiple restorations across different quadrants can be easily performed.
- Patients benefit from the absence of vibrations and odours, fostering maximum cooperation.
- The intermittent, light contact mode facilitates effortless preparation with clear visibility for the dentist.
- Lasers can adeptly navigate curves and folds in the oral cavity, offering versatility in vaporizing, coagulating, or cutting tissue based on power settings and delivery mode.
- Pain is significantly reduced or eliminated in approximately 90% of cases due to the sealing of nerve fibres.
- Lasers minimize the risk of mechanical trauma, such as cracks, reduce bacterial counts, and in some cases, sterilize the operating field.[91]

Limitations

- The primary drawback lies in the cost-effectiveness, as laser treatments tend to be expensive.[91]

- Lasers lack the ability to create intentionally uneven edges, which are necessary for proper retention of dental amalgam or similar materials.

- Laser technology cannot be utilized for repairing existing amalgam fillings due to the vaporization of mercury, resulting in heightened toxicity.

- Another limitation of Erbium family lasers is their inability to remove defective metallic and cast porcelain restorations.

Safety Measures

1) Protective glasses must be worn by everyone in the room, with dark green-tinted glasses recommended for Argon and YAG lasers, and clear glasses for CO2 lasers.

2) Wet gauze pads should be positioned in the patient's mouth around the treated area.

3) Reflective surfaces, such as instruments and mirrors, must be covered to prevent stray light beams from bouncing around the room.

4) Anesthetic gases must be thoroughly removed from the room as they pose an explosive hazard when exposed to laser beams.

5) The dentist should use suction to remove vaporized soft tissue and the smoke or laser plume emitted during procedures, as the plume may carry viruses.

6) Laser treatment is gentle on pulpal tissue and has been shown to have no adverse reactions on pulp health.

6.10 Sonics

Damage to neighbouring tooth surfaces during the completion of proximal cavities is a common occurrence, with smaller cavities often resulting in worse damage. Consequently, efforts have been directed towards developing systems aimed at minimizing iatrogenic damage, particularly in minimally invasive occlusoproximal preparations.

The SONIC flex system by Kavo Dental employs sonic oscillation to cut and refine small proximal cavities. This system utilizes a highly frequent oscillating handpiece, allowing the preparation instruments to transfer their negative form to the tooth. During proximal preparation, damage to neighbouring teeth ranges from 2.5 to 4 bar, with a sonic wave frequency of 6.0 KHz, and the recommended operating pressure is approximately 0.1N.[92,93] The sonic instrumentation facilitates proximal bevelling with minimal risk of damage to adjacent tooth surfaces.

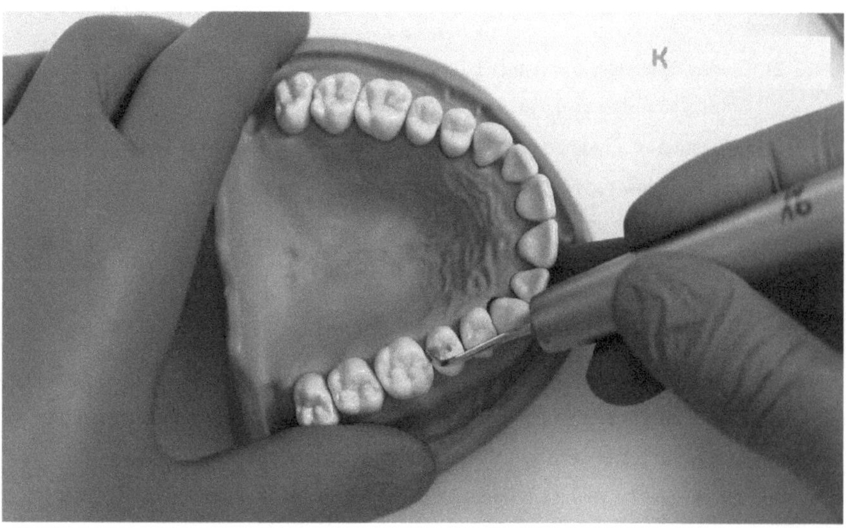

6.11 Ozone therapy

Ozone, a component of the natural gas mix enveloping the Earth at high altitudes, serves as a protective shield against excessive UV radiation for the global population. The refreshing scent often experienced in mountainous regions after thunderstorms is attributed to ozone.

First identified by Schonbein in 1840, ozone (O3) has a significant history of industrial application. Ozone has been employed in the treatment of patients with inflammatory bowel disorders, including ulcerative colitis, Crohn's disease, and chronic bacterial diarrhoea.[94]

Initially, ozone was applied to external body surfaces to assess its effects on various lesions.

Presently, several types of ozone generators are utilized for clinical applications:

1) Production of ozone from oxygen in a narrow frequency band of UV light.

2) Corona discharge, involving a tube with a hot cathode surrounded by a screen anode.

3) Utilization of a method known as 'cold plasma,' which entails a device constructed from two glass rods filled with an inert noble gas excited by high voltage.

The Niche Theory

The development and advancement of caries entail a multifaceted process characterized by the buildup of microorganisms in a specific environment, ultimately resulting in mineral loss from the tooth and the gradual progression of caries throughout the tooth structure. As per the 'niche environment theory,' a distinct 'bacterial niche' forms within a carious lesion.[94]

Mechanism of Action of Ozone

Microbicidal Activity

Ozone's potent biocidal properties stem from its oxidative reactions, which effectively target microorganisms such as bacteria by oxidizing their cell walls and membranes, potentially leading to membrane rupture (Yamayoshi and Tatsumi, 1993). This therapeutic potential of ozone in inhibiting bacterial proliferation was recognized in dentistry as early as 1930.[94,95] Heal ozone harnesses ozone's capabilities to eliminate bacteria, including those implicated in the onset and progression of caries.

Ozone has a long history of use in reducing pathogenic microorganisms (Bocci, 1999; Brauner, 1991). In dentistry, studies have shown significant reductions in C. albicans, methicillin-resistant Staphylococcus aureus (MRSA), and T1 phage after exposure to 10 ppm ozonated water (Murakami et al., 1996). Beyond its antimicrobial effects, ozone has been found to enhance the expression of cytokines crucial for wound healing, exert marked influences on cell proliferation, chemotaxis (of monocytes and fibroblasts), angiogenesis, extracellular matrix synthesis, and collagen synthesis. Ozonated water has proven effective in dental surgery, where it promotes haemostasis, improves local oxygen supply, and inhibits bacterial growth. Gas exposures of 10 and 20 seconds, as well as ozonized water, have demonstrated reductions in cariogenic bacteria (S. mutans and S. sobrinus) (Baysan et al., 2000).

Oxidation of Biomolecules in Dental Diseases

Ozone's potent oxidizing properties not only strip away protein protection and exhibit bactericidal effects but also oxidize the biomolecules essential for sustaining and proliferating the niche (Smith et al., 2001; Claxson et al., 2002; Lynch et al., 2002). Previous studies have demonstrated the remineralizing potential of oxidizing agents, such as sodium hypochlorite. Sodium hypochlorite has proven effective in eliminating organic materials, including proteins, from demineralized dentin, thereby enhancing lesion permeability to fluoride for remineralization (Inaba et al., 1995, 1996). It has been theorized that ozone, being a significantly more potent oxidant than sodium hypochlorite, could similarly remove proteins from carious lesions.

Advantages

1. Absence of injections.
2. Elimination of drilling.
3. Reduction in discomfort.
4. Adoption of conservative preparation methods.
5. Time-saving approach.

Adverse Effects

Excessive concentrations may lead to respiratory distress.

Applications

A. Utilizing Heal Ozone with traditional cups serves as a potent disinfectant before root canal filling during RCT.
B. Effective treatment for Herpes or aphthous ulcers.
C. Application in implant surgeries.
D. Facilitating tooth whitening procedures.
E. Employed in periodontal treatment procedures.

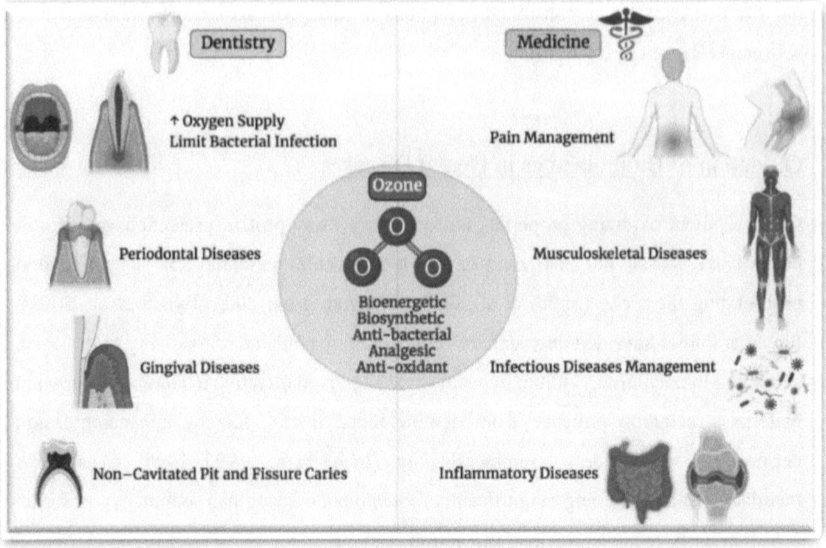

6.12 Genetic modalities in caries prevention

Advanced genetic bioengineering techniques now enable the cloning of genes responsible for cell wall antigens. Recently, researchers have successfully isolated such a gene from S. mutans, inserted it into the DNA of Escherichia coli, and synthesized specific proteins. Similarly, the gene responsible for glucosyl transferase activity has been isolated from S. mutans and inserted into the DNA of E. coli.[96]

In a different approach, Hillman (2002) of Florida has developed an effector strain of Streptococcus mutans, named BCS3-L1, which lacks the lactate dehydrogenase gene. This strain is incapable of producing lactic acid and has been engineered to produce elevated levels of a novel peptide antibiotic called Mutacin 1140.[97] This antibiotic effectively kills conventional S. mutans strains without harming other bacteria.

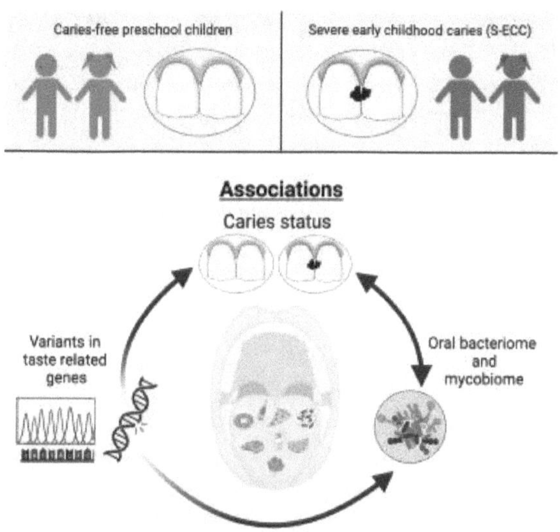

In 1989, Goldberg and Keil achieved successful removal of soft carious dentin using bacterial Achromobacter Collagenase, without impacting the sound layers of dentin beneath the lesion.[98] Similarly, in a study by Norb et al. (1996), the enzyme pronase, a non-specific proteolytic enzyme derived from Streptomyces griseus, was utilized to aid in the removal of soft carious dentin.[99]

RECENT ADVANCES

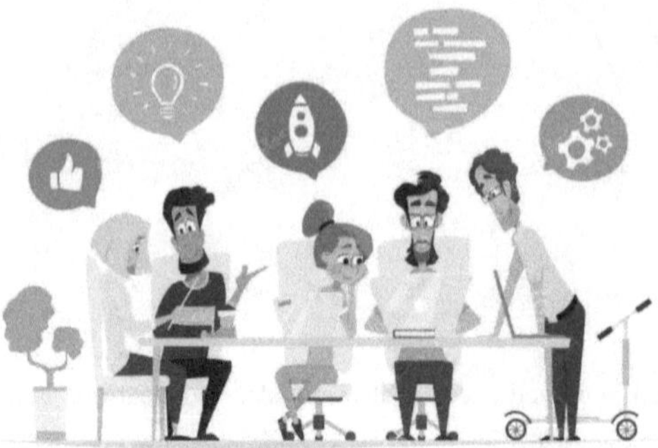

- Microabrasion
- Resin Infilteration
- Bleaching
- Digital Dentistry
- Biomimetic Approach
- Laser assisted techniques
- Nanotechnology

7.1 Microabrasion

This technique, known for its minimally invasive approach, is utilized for the removal of superficial enamel discolorations and imperfections. It is also called as Air abrasion. It entails gently abrading the outer enamel layer using a blend of mild abrasive agents and a high-speed handpiece, as described by Rayapudi and Usha (2018).[100] This method proves highly effective in treating white or brown demineralized spots, fluorosis stains, and mild enamel hypoplasia. Microabrasion offers significant enhancement in the aesthetics of affected teeth without necessitating invasive procedures or extensive tooth preparation. It's often complemented by other minimally invasive methods like enamel bonding or bleaching for achieving optimal outcomes, as highlighted by Kornblit et al. (2008).[100]

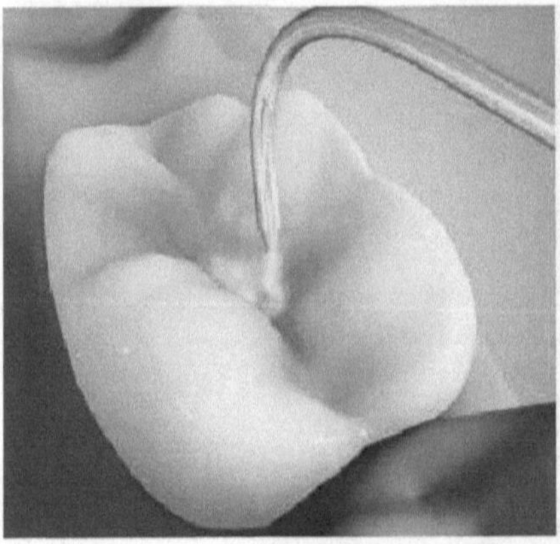

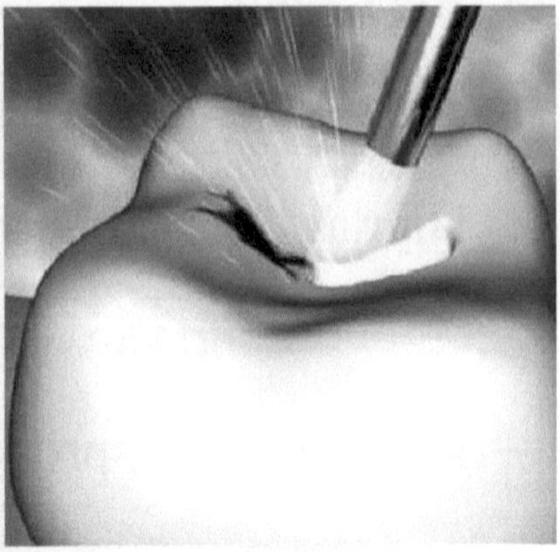

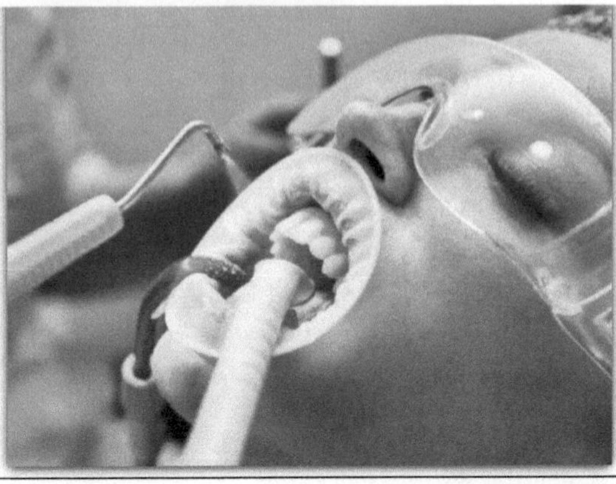

How Does Air Abrasion Work?

In air abrasion, a tool resembling a miniature sandblaster is utilized to eliminate decay. This technique involves directing a fine stream of particles, typically composed of silica, aluminium oxide, or a baking soda mixture, towards the decayed area of the tooth. These particles are propelled towards the tooth surface by compressed air or gas flowing through the dental handpiece. As the stream of particles makes contact with the tooth surface, it effectively removes small particles of decay. Subsequently, the dislodged particles of decay are suctioned away.[26]

Advantages of Air Abrasion:

In comparison to the traditional drilling method, air abrasion offers numerous benefits including:

- Air abrasion does not generate heat, sound, pressure, or vibration.
- Air abrasion diminishes the requirement for anesthesia, especially for shallow cavities.
- Air abrasion preserves a larger portion of healthy tooth tissue.
- Air abrasion keeps the working area relatively dry, which facilitates the placement of composite fillings.
- Air abrasion reduces the risk of micro-fracturing and chipping of the tooth, potentially preventing premature restorative failures.
- Air abrasion enables the dentist to address multiple sites in the mouth during a single visit.
- The procedure is relatively straightforward and expeditious.[26]

Air abrasion also has applications in:

- Eliminating certain old composite restorations, excluding metallic restorations like silver amalgam fillings.
- Preparing tooth surfaces for bonding or sealants.
- Eradicating superficial stains and tooth discolorations.

Drawbacks:[26]

- Air abrasion may not always be entirely painless. Both the air and abrasives employed can induce sensitivity.
- Air abrasion is not advisable for deep cavities located near the tooth's pulp. It is most effective for addressing minor cavities that develop early on the tooth's surface.
- Only composite filling material is compatible with air abrasion, as it adheres effectively to the smooth surface generated by the procedure. Amalgam or silver fillings necessitate drill-based preparations to prevent dislodgement.

7.2 Resin Infiltration

It is employed for the treatment of incipient or non-cavitated carious lesions, particularly those impacting the enamel layer. This procedure entails introducing a low-viscosity resin into the porous enamel structure, effectively halting the advancement of the lesion and enhancing its appearance. By filling the voids within the enamel, the resin infiltrant bolsters its structural integrity while concealing discoloration resulting from carious lesions. This minimally invasive strategy circumvents the removal of healthy tooth structures and serves as an efficient preventive measure against the progression of early-stage caries. Resin infiltration is frequently combined with other minimally invasive restorative approaches to deliver comprehensive care for dental caries, as elucidated by Mirsiaghi et al. (2018).[100]

Indications

1. Small white lesions inherent on the tooth.
2. Decalcified smooth surface white lesion on the tooth such as stasis of plaque after orthodontic treatment, or early smooth surface caries resulting from poor oral hygiene.
3. Larger white marks and bands on the tooth.
4. Molar incisor hypoplasia (MIH).

5. Hypoplasia stains due to traumatic injuries.
6. Mild to moderate fluorosis.
7. Large single bands due to fluorosis.
8. Constructive in arresting of the Non-cavitated Proximal Carious Lesions progression rate.

Contra-indications

1. In the case where patient is allergic to any component of the material used during the procedure.
2. When the carious lesion has extended beyond the outer third of dentin.

Advantages

It is an innovative way of treating initial carious lesions and suits perfectly with the theory of minimal intervention dentistry. It depicts a newer method for the treatment of non-cavitated lesions of proximal and smooth surfaces in primary and permanent teeth up to the first third of dentin (D-1 level).

- Non-invasive treatment, preserving tooth structure.
- Achieved in a single visit.
- Mechanical stabilization of demineralized enamel.
- Arrest/retardation of lesion progress.
- Permanent occlusion of superficial micro-pores and cavities.
- Obturation of porous, deeply demineralized areas.
- Delay of restorative intervention for longer periods.
- Minimized risk of secondary caries.
- No risk of postoperative sensitivity and pulpal Inflammation.
- Reduced risk of gingivitis and periodontitis.
- Improved esthetic outcome when used as a "masking" resin on demineralized labial surfaces (white spot lesions, i.e. with orthodontic patients).
- High patient acceptance.

Disadvantages

- Surface conditioning with 15% hydrochloric acid is necessary because of the presence of hyper mineralised surface layer in initial caries lesions that prohibits the resin to penetrate into the demineralized body of the lesion.

- Resin is extremely hydrophobic. Thus, the resin has to be applied in absolutely dry conditions. Wetness within the body of the lesion or surface of the lesion hampers resin infiltration. Thus, using a rubber dam is necessary.

Technique

Icon® offers two kits: the proximal surface kit and the vestibular surface kit. Both are used similarly, except the proximal kit requires tooth separation. The lesion body has a higher pore volume than the enamel surface layer, forming a barrier to resin infiltration. To prepare the surface, clean and apply 15% hydrochloric acid (Icon Etch) for 2 minutes, stirring occasionally with a micro brush. This acid is superior to 37% phosphoric acid, creating a penetration depth of 58 μm.

Next, desiccate the surface using 99% ethanol (Icon Dry) for 30 seconds followed by air drying. This technique allows hydrophobic monomers to infiltrate demineralized enamel or dentine effectively. Then, apply Icon resin (tetra ethylene glycol dimethacrylate) with a micro brush for about 3 minutes, remove excess material with a cotton roll, and light cure. Repeat for another minute, light cure again, and then polish the surface.

Carefully select cases, as smaller white marks are easier to treat. Medium-to-large patches might need two treatments, and deep lesions may require sandblasting before acid application. Teeth with brown discoloration are not ideal for resin infiltration and might benefit more from micro-abrasion or conventional resin restorations.

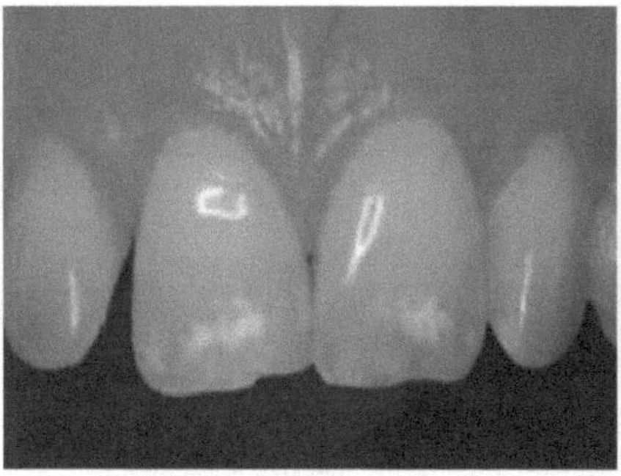

Hypoplastic incisors noted in a patient

1

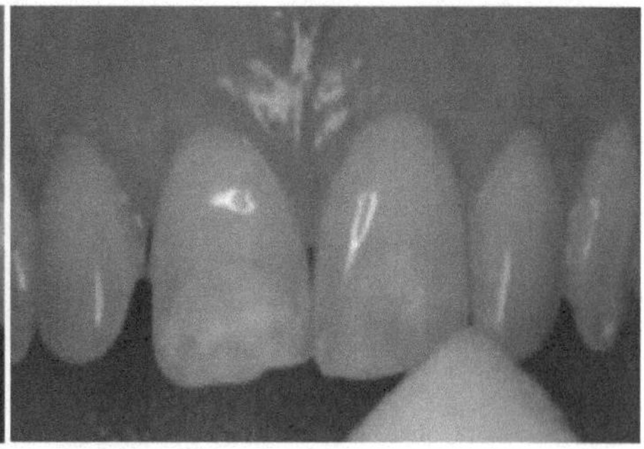

Fig.3. The result after rinsing and air drying.

3

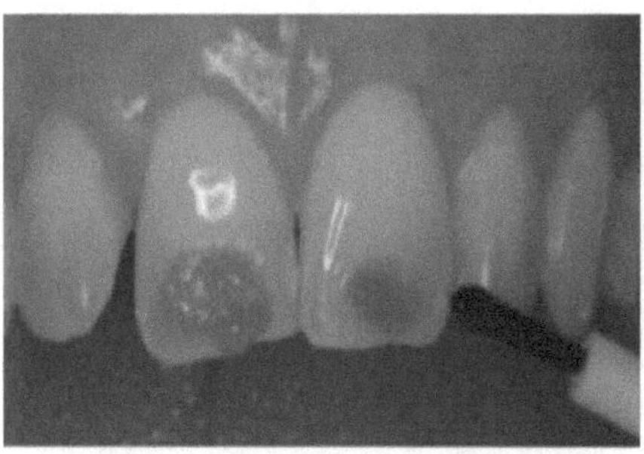

Acid etching with 15% Hydrochloric acid for 2 minutes

2

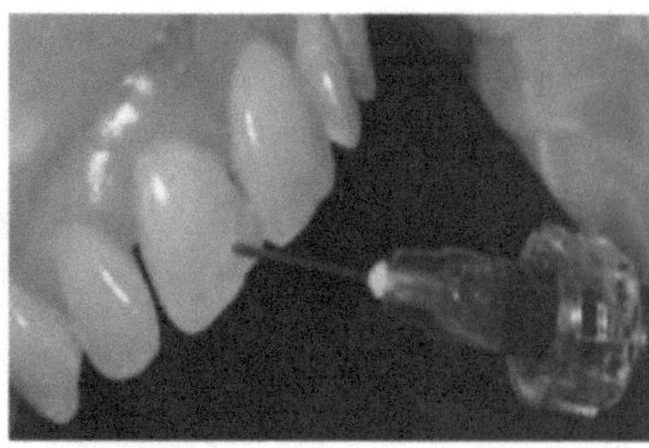

The resin material is injected with a special applicator

4

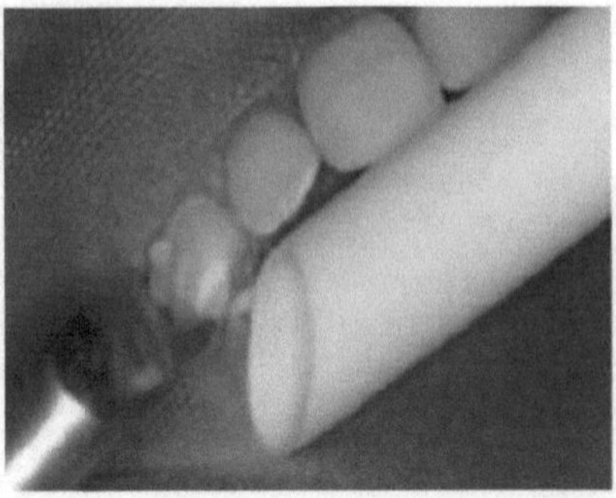

Deeper lesions sandblasted first before etching

5

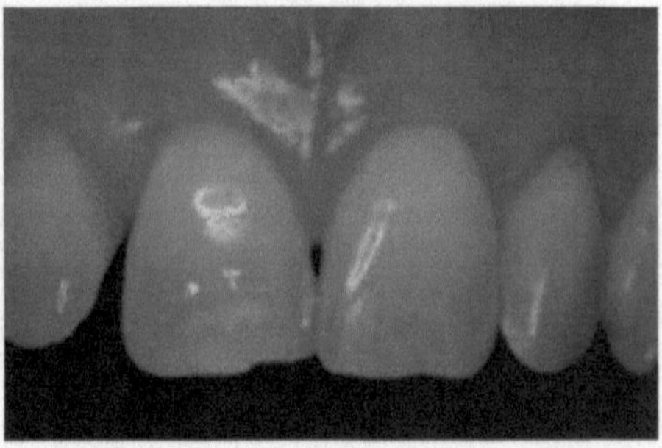

Immediate result after Resin infiltration technique

7

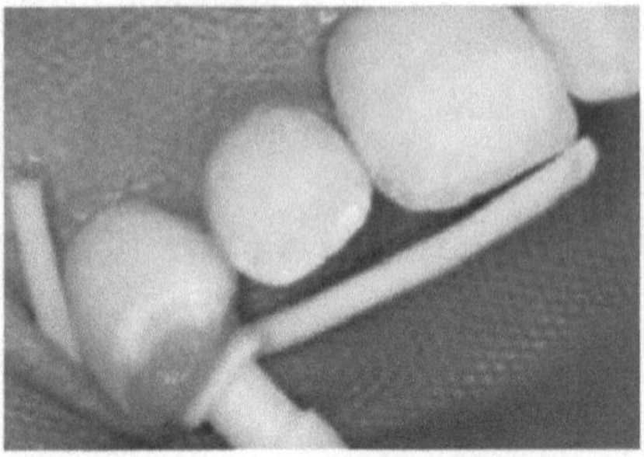

Etching of the tooth after sandblasting process

6

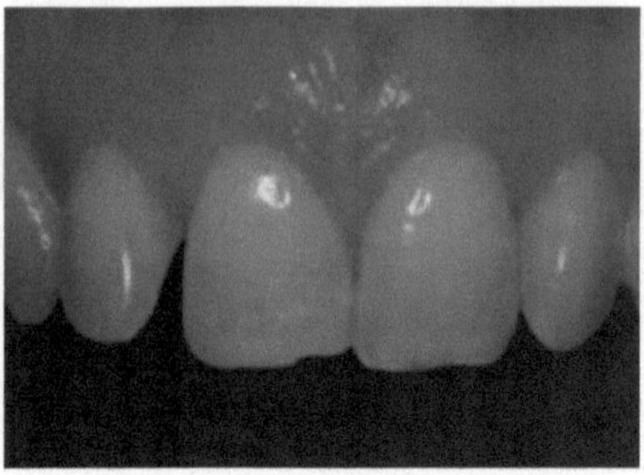

3 Month follow up.

8

Resin infiltration in primary teeth

In primary teeth the progression of proximal caries especially in primary molars is higher when compared to permanent teeth. The mineral composition and the ultra-structure of primary tooth enamel varies with less mineralization and more porous and a prismatic when compares to permanent tooth enamel. Therefore, the diffusion coefficient in primary enamel seems to be greater. The proximal surface layer is less mineralized and thinner in primary molars compared with permanent ones. Thus, etching the surface for 120 seconds with 15% hydrochloric acid in primary teeth, showed reliable and considerable erosion of the mineralized surface layer deeper than that seen in permanent teeth.

Limitations of resin infiltration

Resin infiltration technique has opened up a new range of options for minimal invasive treatment of white spots, yet there are few reasons that may affect the success of the treatment.

- Inefficient isolation.
- Incomplete resin polymerization.
- Depth of the lesion.

7.3 Bleaching

Tooth bleaching stands as a prevalent minimally invasive method aimed at addressing tooth discoloration and elevating smile aesthetics. This technique entails the application of bleaching agents like hydrogen peroxide or carbamide peroxide to eliminate intrinsic and extrinsic stains from the tooth's structure. Bleaching can be conducted either in a professional setting under supervision or at home utilizing custom trays and bleaching gels. This method proves effective in enhancing the shade and luminosity of teeth without necessitating invasive procedures. It proves particularly advantageous for individuals with tooth discoloration stemming from aging, tobacco use, or specific dietary habits. Bleaching presents a conservative and economically viable approach to enhancing smile aesthetics and can be synergistically employed with other minimally invasive procedures such as micro abrasion or composite resin restorations for comprehensive outcomes, as discussed by Prabhakar et al. (2015).[100]

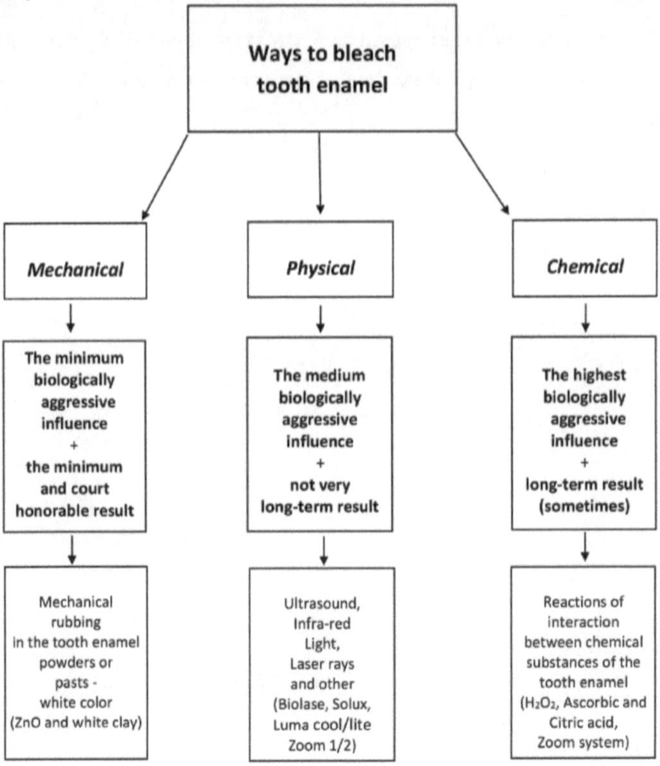

7.4 Digital dentistry and Computer-aided design/computer-aided manufacturing (CAD/CAM) technology

Computer-aided design (CAD) refers to the practice of creating a digital 3D model of a dental product with software, as opposed to a traditional wax-up. Computer-aided manufacturing (CAM) refers to techniques like CNC milling and 3D printing that are done by machines and controlled by software, as opposed to traditional processes like casting or ceramic layering, which are entirely manual. It describes the use of CAD tools and CAM methods to produce crowns, dentures, inlays, onlays, bridges, veneers, implants, and abutment restorations or prostheses. This technology allows for the accurate crafting of restorations, diminishing reliance on conventional impressions and simplifying the process of planning minimally invasive treatments (Kumar et al., 2021).[100] In the simplest terms, a dentist or technician would use CAD software to create the virtual crown, for example, which would be manufactured with a CAM process. As you can imagine, CAD/CAM dentistry is more replicable and scalable than conventional methods.

Advantages of CAD/CAM dentistry

The biggest advantage of CAD/CAM dentistry is speed. These techniques can deliver a dental product in as little as one day and sometimes the same day if the dentist designs and manufactures in house. It also allows dental labs to finish far more products per day with less effort and fewer manual steps. Because CAD/CAM dentistry is faster and has a simpler workflow, it is also more cost-effective for dental practices and labs. CAD/CAM dentistry typically requires fewer patient visits, too one for the intra-oral scan and one for placement which is much more convenient. It is also more comfortable for patients because they can be scanned digitally and avoid the unpleasant process of holding a viscous wad of alginate in their mouth for up to five minutes while it sets. Product quality is also higher with CAD/CAM dentistry. The digital accuracy of intraoral scanners, 3D design software, milling machines and 3D printers often produces more predictable results that fit patients more accurately. CAD/CAM dentistry has also made it possible for practices to handle complex restorations more easily.

Applications of CAD/CAM dentistry

The applications of CAD/CAM dentistry are primarily in restorative work, or the repair and replacement of teeth that have decay, damage, or are missing. CAD/CAM technology can be used to create a wide range of dental products, including Crowns, Inlays, Onlays, Veneers, Bridges, Full and partial dentures, Implant restorations. Overall, CAD/CAM dentistry is appealing because it is faster and easier while frequently delivering better results.

7.5 Biomimetic approaches

Biomimetic dentistry strives to replicate the inherent structure and functionality of teeth through materials and methodologies that closely emulate natural tooth properties, leading to improved durability and aesthetics (Da Mata et al., 2015).[100]

Biomimetic Restorative Dentistry

The main objective of biomimetic restorative dentistry is to return the hard tissues (enamel, dentin, cementum) to attain full function through a restorative material that can mimic or restore the biomechanics of the natural tooth. This allows the tooth to function as one unit against functional forces and provides near normal biology, and aesthetics.

- In conventional extension for prevention approach, not only the diseased but also sound tooth structure are removed and replaced with rigid, non-responsive materials. This treatment plan usually weakens the remaining tooth structure and yields a short life span restoration.

- In Biomimetic approach, the concept of less or no dentistry is the best dentistry has been adopted. It is conservative and only focuses on restoring the teeth and simulating the natural dentition as much as possible. The biomimetic restorative protocols aim to achieve these results by stress-reducing protocols and bond-maximizing protocols. Cavities and other lesions are carefully repaired using advanced materials and adhesives so the tooth retains its inherent natural properties.

Biomimetic restorative materials

1. Glass Ionomer Cement (Man-made dentin)

It is the generic name of a group of materials that use silicate glass powder and aqueous solution of polyacrylic acid. They undergo a significant acid—base reaction as a part of their setting reaction and show a continuing fluoride release. Glass ionomer cements (GICs) are considered as biomimetic materials because they have the same coefficient of thermal expansion as that of tooth structure, bond adhesively to enamel and dentin, and release fluoride over a prolonged period of time. GIC's ability to release ions is responsible for the development of long-term durable bonds at the tooth/restoration interface. Studies have shown that ions can move from the cement and from the tooth into the interfacial region to create an ion-exchange layer that proved to be highly durable in clinical service. In spite of these advantages, conventional glass ionomers suffer from disadvantages such as short working times, long setting times, brittleness, low fracture toughness, and susceptibility to moisture contamination or dehydration during the early stages of the setting reaction. Various modifications in the powder and liquid of glass ionomer material have been done to improve its performance.

Nano-hydroxyapatite (HA) particles have been added to GIC to produce GIC-HA hybrids, which showed improved release of fluoride ions, and improved mechanical and antibacterial properties. Moreover, Garoushi et al. in a recent study explored the effect of addition of hollow and solid discontinuous glass fiber fillers on fracture toughness and flexural strength of GIC and resin modified GICs. Results showed significant enhancement in fracture toughness (280 and 200%) and flexural strength (170 and 140%) of hollow discontinuous glass fiber (10 wt. %) added to GICs.

In 2020, Singer et al. modified the antimicrobial activity of GIC with a mixture of three natural plant extracts (Salvadora persica, Olea europaea, and Ficus carcia). The three plant extracts improved the antimicrobial activity against S. mutans and against M. luteus while compressive strength was improved by addition of the plant extracts at higher concentrations.

2. Dental composite resin

Nearly everything in nature, including teeth, pearls, shells, corals, and bones, is composed of hybrid organic and inorganic composites with the structures of each component regulating the final performance of the hybrids. Dental composite resin (DCR) represents an important category of hybrid biomaterials, which are composed of a resin matrix and inorganic fillers. DCR has been widely applied in dentistry to restore diseased and defective teeth since the 1960s because of their excellent aesthetics, good biocompatibility, and ease of use.

Self-healing/Bleeding material is a resin composite system, which employs a biomimetic approach to perform a self-repairing function. Many natural materials are themselves self-healing composites as the natural bone, which has the ability to self-heal even with major fracture. Self-healing could be either intrinsic or extrinsic, according to whether the reparative molecules are produced only in response to damage (intrinsic) or are already deposited within the material (extrinsic).

Intrinsic self-healing occurs at the molecular level, and an external source of energy is required to control the movement of the reactants. On the other hand, extrinsic self-healing materials usually rely on polymeric capsules, which rupture near the crack and release the resin that reacts with an existing catalyst resulting in polymerization of the resin and crack repair. Visual enhancement of the damage could be achieved as well by the bleeding of a highly added conspicuous medium such as fluorescent dye.

Bilayered resin composite structure is considered a new biomimetic restoration system, which mimics the fibrous structure of dentin-enamel complex. It is made of a base formed of glass fiber reinforced composite resin (FRC) and a surface of a more polishable and wear resistant resin composite. The function of the FRC base for filling composites is to provide a crack propagation prevention layer for the restoration.

3. Ceramics

Dental ceramics are able to mimic the natural appearance of the tooth. The popularity of dental ceramics has been widely extended in the last three decades after the evolution in computer based dental technologies and the introduction of the "digital workflow" concept in dentistry. In 2000, Holland et al. were able to develop an apatite-leucite glass ceramics that are made of needle-like apatite building blocks similar to those found in the living dental tissues. The needle-like apatite crystals improved the esthetic and mechanical properties of the material. Biomimetic dental ceramics should be able to establish gap free adhesion to the restored dental substance and to promote natural regeneration of surrounding tissues. Goudouri et al. succeeded to incorporate an apatite-forming ability to a commercial dental restorative ceramic material to enhance the tissue attachment. The specimens demonstrated the formation of apatite-like layer on the surface without affecting the flexural strength of the material. Several bioactive glass–ceramics are commercially available and were used to coat titanium and zirconia dental implants. The coating enhanced the Osseo integration and tissue bonding around ceramic implants.

Hybrid ceramics are another example of biomimetic ceramic materials. They were introduced in a trial to combine the advantages of ceramics and composites in order to get physical properties (e.g., Youngs modulus and hardness) similar to that of enamel and dentin. Recently, researchers of material science have developed functionally graded polymers infiltrated ceramic network that are characterized by gradients in composition and structure to produce a structure that have properties of enamel and dentine combined.

Since the tooth is made up of different structures (enamel and dentin) which have different optical and physical properties, the possibility of mimicking both tissues with one layer of material is not an easy task. Furthermore, the concept of biomimetics was recently extended to include gradients in strength within the same ceramic block. A novel multilayered zirconia block that integrates different types of zirconia together in one block was introduced. These new blocks are monolithic restorations that contains yttria partially stabilized tetragonal zirconia polycrystal (3Y-TZP) in the body area to provide high mechanical stability and 5Y-TZP in the occlusal area to provide the desired aesthetics.

Biomimetic Regenerative Dentistry

Dentin remineralisation

Demineralisation is the process of removing mineral ions from Hydroxyapatite (HA) crystals of enamel, dentin, cementum, and bone. Depositing lost mineral ions again to the demineralized crystals is called remineralization. Considerable number of mineral ions could be lost from HA without destroying its integrity but high sensitivity to heat, cold, pressure, and pain would be expected which is termed dentin hypersensitivity. Once the integrity of HA crystal lattice becomes lost, dental cavities can be clearly seen. Demineralisation is not an irreversible process; hence, the demineralized HA crystals can grow back to their original size under favourable remineralisation conditions.

1. Crystallite's growth conventional remineralisation approach

Conventional remineralisation protocols of the carious dentin often involve using formulations with calcium and phosphate ions of different concentrations. In this case, remineralisation occurs by epitaxial growth of residual apatite crystals in partially demineralized dentin rather than new crystals nucleation. If there are no or very few residual crystals, there will be no remineralisation. The mineral content of the surface layer of the lesion affects the quality of the resulting remineralisation, including its location and mineral deposition density.

2. Bottom-up biomimetic remineralisation approaches

The biomimetic remineralisation process is a bottom-up approach used to create nanocrystals that are small enough to fit in the gaps between adjacent collagen molecules in order to backfill the demineralized dentin collagen. These nano precursor particles (amorphous calcium phosphate (ACP) nano-precursors) are stabilized by biomimetic analogues of non-collagenous proteins (dentin matrix protein (DMP1) and dentin phosphophoryn (DPP, DMP2) that regulate the HA crystal nucleation growth. In this direction, several bioactive materials and non-collagenous proteins (NCPs) analogues have been used to promote remineralisation.

Biomimetic dentin remineralisation materials

Bioactive materials

1. Bioactive Glass
2. Casein phosphopeptide–amorphous calcium phosphate (CPP-ACP)
3. Fluoride compounds
4. Zinc oxide loaded materials

7.6 Laser-assisted techniques

Dental lasers offer accurate and minimally intrusive treatment alternatives for a range of procedures, such as cavity preparation, soft tissue management, and tooth whitening (Banerjee, 2015).[100]

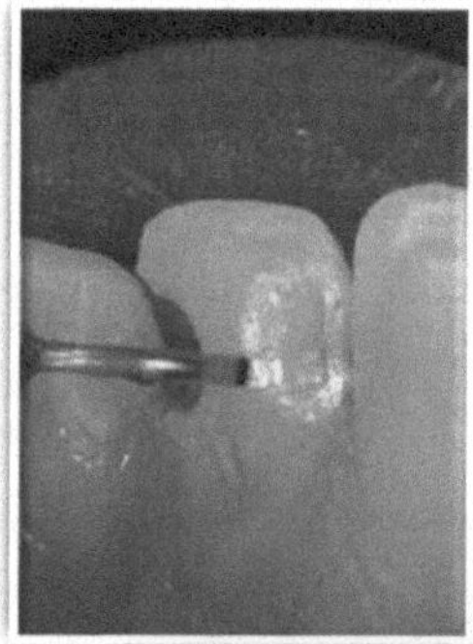

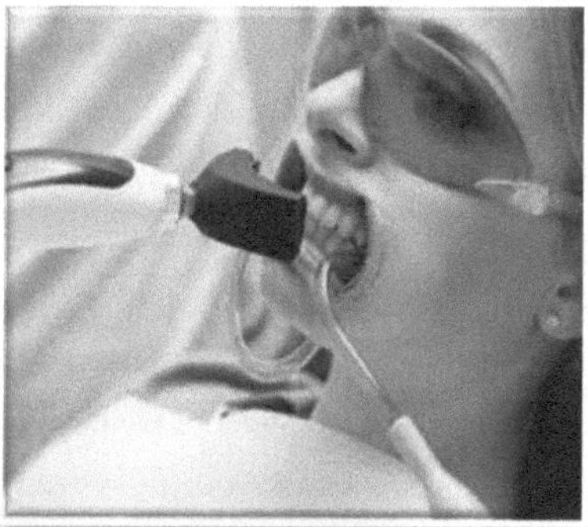

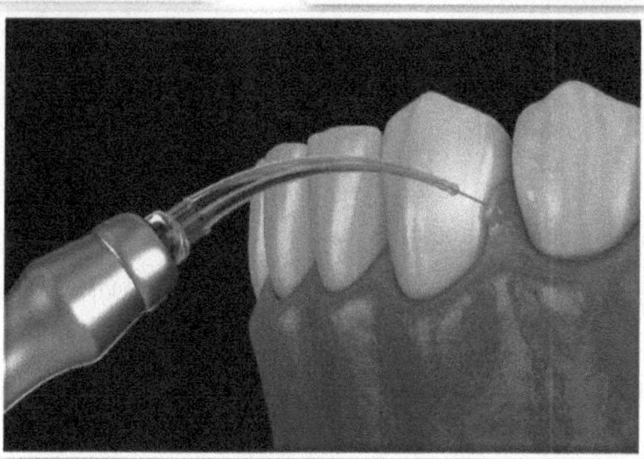

7.7 Nanotechnology

Nano-materials are used to manipulate materials on an atomic or molecular level. However, on a nanoscale, the chemical, biological, and physical properties of an atom vary compared to its naturally occurring compound forms. Human tooth structures include enamel that is made of 96% hydroxyapatite of size ranging from 10nm to 200 nm. Intertubular dentin is 2-5nm in thickness and 60nm in length. Enamel and dentin are connected by collagen fibrils that stretch over 20-75 nm in length. These characteristics provide a solid ground for the basic need for research applications of nano-materials in dentistry. Nanomaterials provide enhanced physical and mechanical attributes, allowing for the development of stronger and aesthetically pleasing restorations with minimal tooth preparation (Tumenas et al., 2014).[100] The use of nano-materials in dentistry is known as nano dentistry.

A wide variety of materials are available to restore the lost form and function of decayed teeth. Use of conventional dental amalgam was widely in use as restorative material in stress bearing areas due to its superior strength, but has compromised aesthetics due to its metallic color. Esthetic demands have necessitated the use of tooth coloured restorative materials like dental composites and glass-ionomer cements. Though they are superior as esthetic restorative materials in anterior tooth region, they could not effectively bear the occlusal forces in the posterior regions. Incorporation of nano particles into these materials has enhanced the physical properties and favoured the use of these materials in the posterior tooth region. This led to the development of materials like nano-composites, nano-bonding systems, nano-GIC, nano-varnish and sealants.

Nano-composites

Nanocomposites are available as nanofills (1-100 nm) and nanohybrids (0.4-5 μm). Nanofillers include nanomeric particles or nanoclusters like monodispersed colloidal silica. These are typically invisible, not affecting optical properties. They enhance resin mechanical strength with increased volume. Nanofills combine nano- and micro sized fillers for materials like 3M Filtek. Nanoclusters like zirconia-silica or silica treated with

3-methacryloxypropyltrimethoxysilane (0.6 µm) offer alternatives. Ceramic nanofillers are studied for aesthetics and durability. Carbon nanotubes provide good mechanical properties and bioactivity. Restorative materials incorporate anti-caries properties with remineralizing or anti-cariogenic materials like nanoparticles of dicalcium phosphate anhydrous, nano-hydroxyapatite, and nano-acidulated calcium phosphates. Nanobioglass aids fluoride release. Nano particles such as chlorhexidine and quaternary ammonium compounds are effective for anti-cariogenic properties.

Nano-Bonding system

Incorporation of nano-particles in dentin bonding agents have shown to improve tubular penetration and thereby increasing the mechanical properties of the restoration (e.g. : prime & bond NT, Dentsply). Nano silver particles, Nano amorphous calcium phosphate and Nano quaternary ammonium dimethacrylate (nQADM) are few of the widely studied materials. Recently Colloidal platinum nanoparticles have shown to increase the bond strength of resin. Similarly, Spherical zirconia nanoparticles are used in bonding systems which aids in stabilizing the hybrid layer. Newly, the concept of nanogels has been introduced. They are 10- to 100-nm particles which on interaction with monomers get swollen. This property allows penetration of adhesives deep into dentin and increase the bond strength.

Nano-GIC

Wilson and Kent in 1971 introduced GIC, ever since it has been a widely used in dentistry like Ketac Nano (3m ESPE). But, it had lower mechanical properties than other traditional restorative materials. The incorporation of nanoparticles favoured to increase particle size distribution and thereby increasing the mechanical values of GIC. Forsterite nanoparticles, when incorporated in GIC enhanced the fluoride release. Nano-fluorapatite or nano fluoro hydroxyapatite has also showed similar properties. Use of nano agglomerated glass has improved the compressive strength if GIC. Recently, resin modified glass ionomers are modified by addition of nanoparticles and nanoclusters in fluoro-aluminosilicate glass. It resulted in the aesthetic improvement of the final restoration and polishablilty. It has led to the improvement is setting reaction, Improvement in poly salt bridge formation, Better bonding with dentin and More compressive strength. Similarly, Nanoparticles of CHX hexametaphosphate are used as an anti-microbial agent but nano-chlorhexidine modified GIC shows less fluoride release than conventional one which is a drawback.

Nano-Varnish and sealants

Hydroxyapatite and fluorapatite bioceramic nano-fibers have nanostructure solubility which aids in effective release of fluorine ions. Which when incorporated in sealant system can cause caries prevention. The nano-sealants provide wear resistance and a reduced shrinkage. Another application of nanotechnology is the development of a nano-filled light curing varnish. It is used to protect GIC during early maturation phase. It prevents water sorption ad dehydration of GIC thereby, improving its mechanical properties. E.g., EQUIA ('Easy-Quick- Unique-Intelligent-Aesthetic').

Nano coating of restorations

Nano-filled, light-cured preparations are used as a protective coating for composite and acrylic indirect composites like the Optiglaze Glossy Protective Coating Agent (GC Corporation, Japan). These solutions provide an aesthetic glossy surface and can be used in difficult to polish areas such as posterior fissures or interproximal areas of indirect composite restorations. It can be used on indirect composite restorations, artificial teeth, removable dentures, temporary crowns and individual acrylic trays to provide a glossy finish.

Nano polishing system

Polishing of dental surfaces is a known practice in dentistry which is used to make it difficult for plaque and cariogenic bacteria to accumulate on tooth surfaces. Micron-sized silica particles are a typical component of conventional polishing pastes. The smaller the abrasive particle size the smoother the polished surface. Chemical-mechanical planarization process is one such approach, used in the semiconductor industry which uses various nanometre-sized particles to polish surfaces of semi-conductor wafers to a sub-nanometre level. This was adopted to polish dental surfaces by R.M. Gaikwad and I. Sokolov (2008), where they have used silver nano particles and demonstrated that it is easier to remove bacteria from areas polished with silica nanoparticles. And it can be used for dental polishing.

Nano ceramics

With the integration of nanotechnology and ceramics a new CAD/CAM block of monolithic esthetic material was developed as Lava Ultimate (3M ESPE). It is a mix of nano particles agglomerated in clusters and individual bonded nano particles embedded in a highly cross-linked polymer matrix. The main advantage of this material is said to be the easier clinical finishing and polishing, without the need for a porcelain oven, with the strength, surface gloss and finish retention similar to ceramic materials which has been the main limitation of composite blocks. Its typical composition is made up of non-agglomerated/non-aggregated silica (20 nm), aggregated zirconia (4 to 11 nm particles) or silica clusters (20 nm particles) and non-agglomerated or non-aggregated zirconia (4 to 11 nm) with approximately an 80% ceramic load. A nano optimized mouldable ceramics are developed recently and marketed by the name XircOn Ultra, which is approved by FDA. It is a hybrid nano-ceramic that can bend and flex in the mouth. It is made by a combination of nano-ceramics and polymers. It is said to be one of the closest material to human teeth. Nano fillers enhance polishability reduce wear. The use of nano pigments adjust the shade of the restoration by chameleon effect and nano modifiers increases the stability of the material thereby prevent sticking to instruments. With evolution of material science, newer dental materials are being developed for improving the ease of use and mechanical properties. Nanotechnology is playing a key role in such product development and has proven to be an efficient method for this purpose. A thorough knowledge of these nano restorative materials and its applications helps in efficient use in dentistry. In future, the use of nano-robots seems to be the effective way in restoring early tooth surface defects and carious lesions. But it is still a clinically unexplored arena and the wait doesn't seem too far to explore it.

FUTURE TRENDS

Potential advancements and innovations

The realm of minimally invasive dentistry is in a state of continuous evolution, with several potential advancements and innovations on the horizon. These include:

1. Advancements in restorative materials

Persistent research efforts are directed towards the development of novel restorative materials boasting enhanced durability, aesthetics, and biocompatibility. Biomimetic materials, such as bioactive composites and smart materials, are being investigated for their potential in minimally invasive restorations, aiming to closely replicate the natural properties of teeth (Whitehouse, 2004).

2. Digital Dentistry and three-dimensional (3D printing)

The integration of digital dentistry and 3D printing technology presents promising prospects for minimally invasive dentistry. CAD and CAM systems, coupled with 3D printing, facilitate precise fabrication of restorations, thereby improving accuracy, efficiency, and customization (Cullum and Deporter, 2015).

3. Regenerative approaches

Regenerative techniques, such as stem cell therapies and tissue engineering, hold the potential to regenerate damaged or lost dental tissues. These approaches may revolutionize restorative dentistry by fostering natural healing and regeneration of tooth structures, thus reducing the necessity for invasive interventions (Manaia et al., 2021).

4. Minimally invasive implant dentistry

Advancements in implant dentistry are concentrated on the development of minimally invasive techniques for implant placement and restoration. Techniques such as guided implant surgery, immediate implant loading, and innovative implant materials are being explored to optimize treatment outcomes while minimizing invasiveness (Nguyen et al., 2022).

SUMMARY

Minimally invasive dentistry has revolutionized the way paediatric dental care is approached, offering a more conservative and patient-friendly alternative to traditional methods. This approach prioritizes the preservation of healthy tooth structure while effectively treating dental issues in children. By intervening early and using techniques that minimize the removal of tooth material, paediatric dentists can address problems with minimal discomfort and trauma for the child. The future of minimally invasive dentistry in paediatric dentistry looks promising due to ongoing advancements in various aspects such as materials, technology, and behavioral management techniques. For instance, there are continuous developments in dental materials that allow for more conservative restorations, reducing the need for extensive drilling and preserving more of the natural tooth. Additionally, advancements in technology, such as laser dentistry and digital imaging, provide more precise and minimally invasive treatment options.

Furthermore, behavioral management strategies play a crucial role in minimizing the stress and anxiety associated with dental visits for children. Techniques such as tell-show-do, distraction techniques, and positive reinforcement help create a comfortable environment, ensuring children feel at ease during dental procedures. By effectively managing behavior, paediatric dentists can enhance treatment outcomes and promote positive dental experiences for young patients. Continued research is essential for further refining and validating minimally invasive techniques in paediatric dentistry. Long-term clinical studies, comparative effectiveness research, and ongoing development of materials are vital for establishing evidence-based protocols and improving treatment outcomes. This ongoing research ensures that paediatric dentists have access to the most effective and least invasive techniques to provide the best possible care for their young patients.

By embracing the principles of minimally invasive dentistry and integrating advancements in materials, technology, and behavioral management, paediatric dental professionals can offer conservative yet effective care. This approach leads to improved oral health outcomes, enhanced patient comfort, and increased satisfaction for both children and their families, ultimately promoting better overall oral health in the paediatric population.

"Minimally invasive dentistry teaches us that even the smallest interventions can lead to significant improvements, much like how small, consistent efforts can create profound changes in our lives."

REFERENCES

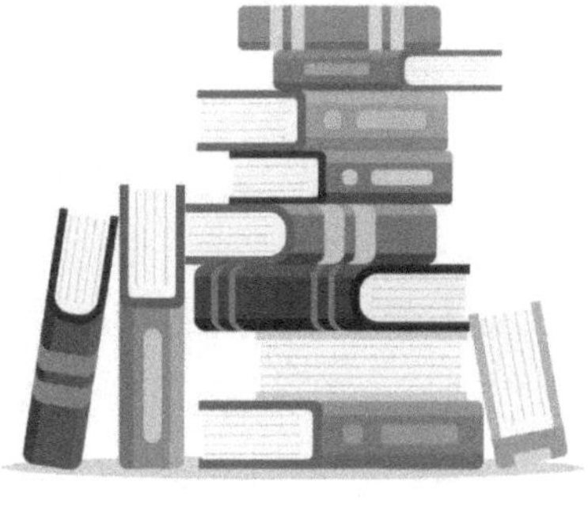

1. Frencken JE, Peters MC, Manton DJ, Leal SC, Gordan VV, Eden E. Minimal intervention dentistry for managing dental caries – a review. International Dental Journal. 2012 Oct;62(5):223–43.

2. Bhatiya P, Thosar N. Minimal invasive dentistry – An emerging trend in pediatric dentistry: A review. International Journal of Contemporary Dental and Medical Reviews. 2015 Feb 27;Article ID 320115:6 pages.

3. Mondal DrA, Pradhan DrS, Chakrabarty DrS. Minimally invasive dentistry a short review of the concepts. IJRTI. 2023 Aug;8(8):608–15.

4. International Caries Detection and Assessment System (ICDAS): A New Concept - PMC [Internet]. [cited 2024 Mar 2].

5. Marwah N. Minimal intervention. Textbook of Pediatric Dentistry. 2nd ed. New Delhi: Jaypee Brothers Medical Publishers. 2009:450-5.

6. Mount GJ, Tyas JM, Duke ES, Hume WR, Lasfargues JJ, Kaleka R. A proposal for a new classification of lesions of exposed tooth surfaces. Int Dent J. 2006 Apr;56(2):82–91.

7. Guideline on caries-risk assessment and management for infants, children, and adolescents - PubMed [Internet]. [cited 2024 Jan 25].

8. Mm J, Nk B, A P. Minimal intervention dentistry - a new frontier in clinical dentistry. J Clin Diagn Res. 2014 Jul;8(7):ZE04-08.

9. van Loveren C, Duggal MS. The role of diet in caries prevention. Int Dent J. 2001;51(6 Suppl 1):399–406.

10. Mickenautsch S, Leal SC, Yengopal V, Bezerra AC, Cruvinel V. Sugar-free chewing gum and dental caries: a systematic review. J Appl Oral Sci. 2007 Apr;15(2):83–8.

11. Carvalho JC, Ekstrand KR, Thylstrup A. Dental plaque and caries on occlusal surfaces of first permanent molars in relation to stage of eruption. J Dent Res. 1989 May;68(5):773–9.

12. Griffin SO, Oong E, Kohn W, Vidakovic B, Gooch BF, CDC Dental Sealant Systematic Review Work Group, et al. The effectiveness of sealants in managing caries lesions. J Dent Res. 2008 Feb;87(2):169–74.

13. Whelton H, O'Mullane D. The use of combinations of caries preventive procedures. J Dent Educ. 2001 Oct;65(10):1110–3.

14. Simratvir M, Singh N, Chopra S, Thomas AM. Efficacy of 10% Povidone Iodine in children affected with early childhood caries: an in vivo study. J Clin Pediatr Dent. 2010;34(3):233–8.

15. Yengopal V. Essential oils for caries prevention: a viable option? SADJ. 2004 Sep;59(8):337, 339–40.

16. Vinod D, Gopalakrishnan A, Subramani SM, Balachandran M, Manoharan V, Joy A. A Comparative Evaluation of Remineralizing Potential of Three Commercially Available Remineralizing Agents: An In Vitro Study. Int J Clin Pediatr Dent. 2020;13(1):61–5.

17. Azrak B, Callaway A, Knözinger S, Willershausen B. Reduction of the pH-values of whole saliva after the intake of apple juice containing beverages in children and adults. Oral Health Prev Dent. 2003;1(3):229–36.

18. Yamazaki H, Litman A, Margolis HC. Effect of fluoride on artificial caries lesion progression and repair in human enamel: regulation of mineral deposition and dissolution under in vivo-like conditions. Arch Oral Biol. 2007 Feb;52(2):110–20.

19. Vashisht R, Kumar A, Indira R, Srinivasan MR, Ramachandran S. Remineralization of early enamel lesions using casein phosphopeptide amorphous calcium Phosphate: an ex-vivo study. Contemp Clin Dent. 2010 Oct;1(4):210–3.

20. Reynolds EC. Calcium phosphate-based remineralization systems: scientific evidence? Aust Dent J. 2008 Sep;53(3):268–73.

21. (PDF) Remineralization of early caries lesions with glass ionomer cements [internet]. [cited 2024 jan 25].

22. Staehle HJ. Minimally invasive restorative treatment. J Adhes Dent. 1999;1(3):267–84.

23. Taifour D, Frencken JE, Beiruti N, van 't Hof MA, Truin GJ. Effectiveness of glass-ionomer (ART) and amalgam restorations in the deciduous dentition: results after 3 years. Caries Res. 2002;36(6):437–44.

24. Morrow LA, Hassall DC, Watts DC, Wilson NH. A chemomechanical method for caries removal. Dent Update. 2000 Oct;27(8):398–401.

25. Minimal Intervention in Pediatric Dentistry | Journal of Orofacial Research [Internet]. [cited 2024 Jan 25].

26. Hegde VS, Khatavkar RA. A new dimension to conservative dentistry: Air abrasion. J Conserv Dent. 2010 Jan;13(1):4–8.

27. Kotlow L. Lasers and pediatric dental care. Gen Dent. 2008;56(7):618–27.

28. Innes NP, Evans DJP, Stirrups DR. The Hall Technique; a randomized controlled clinical trial of a novel method of managing carious primary molars in general dental practice: acceptability of the technique and outcomes at 23 months. BMC Oral Health. 2007 Dec 20;7:18.

29. Mount GJ, Ngo H. Minimal intervention: a new concept for operative dentistry. Quintessence Int. 2000 Sep;31(8):527–33.

30. Sandeep k, sadik m, martha s. Minimal invasive dentistry. 2022.

31. Histological Validation of Electrical Resistance Measurements in the Diagnosis of Occlusal Caries | Caries Research | Karger Publishers [Internet]. [cited 2024 Jan 29].

32. Electrical Conductance and Electrode Area on Sound Smooth Enamel in Extracted Teeth | Caries Research | Karger Publishers [Internet]. [cited 2024 Jan 29].

33. Ekstrand KR, Ricketts DN, Kidd EA, Qvist V, Schou S. Detection, diagnosing, monitoring and logical treatment of occlusal caries in relation to lesion activity and

severity: an in vivo examination with histological validation. Caries Res. 1998;32(4):247–54.

34. Validity of Electrical Conductance Measurements in Evaluating the Marginal Integrity of Sealant Restorations | Caries Research | Karger Publishers [Internet]. [cited 2024 Jan 29].

35. Ie YL, Verdonschot EH, Schaeken MJ, van't Hof MA. Electrical conductance of fissure enamel in recently erupted molar teeth as related to caries status. Caries Res. 1995;29(2):94–9.

36. Posteruptive changes of electrical resistance values in fissure enamel of premolars - PubMed [Internet]. [cited 2024 Jan 29].

37. Ricketts DNJ, Kidd EAM, Wilson RF. The Effect of Airflow on Site-Specific Electrical Conductance Measurements Used in the Diagnosis of Pit and Fissure Caries in vitro. Caries Research. 2009 Nov 24;31(2):111–8.

38. In vivo Diagnosis of Fissure Caries Using a New Electrical Resistance Monitor | Caries Research | Karger Publishers [Internet]. [cited 2024 Jan 29].

39. Detection of dental decay and its extent using a.c. impedence spectroscopy | Nature Medicine [Internet]. [cited 2024 Jan 29].

40. Ricketts DN, Kidd EA, Wilson RF. Electronic diagnosis of occlusal caries in vitro: adaptation of the technique for epidemiological purposes. Community Dent Oral Epidemiol. 1997 Jun;25(3):238–41.

41. Surface-specific electrical occlusal caries diagnosis: reproducibility, correlation with histological lesion depth, and tooth type dependence - PubMed [Internet]. [cited 2024 Jan 29].

42. Huysmans MC, Longbottom C, Pitts NB, Los P, Bruce PG. Impedance spectroscopy of teeth with and without approximal caries lesions--an in vitro study. J Dent Res. 1996 Nov;75(11):1871–8.

43. Human teeth with and without dental caries studied by visible luminescent spectroscopy - PubMed [Internet]. [cited 2024 Jan 29].

44. Bjelkhagen H, Sundström F, Angmar-Månsson B, Rydén H. Early detection of enamel caries by the luminescence excited by visible laser light. Swed Dent J. 1982;6(1):1–7.

45. de Josselin de Jong E, Sundström F, Westerling H, Tranaeus S, ten Bosch JJ, Angmar-Månsson B. A new method for in vivo quantification of changes in initial enamel caries with laser fluorescence. Caries Res. 1995;29(1):2–7.

46. al-Khateeb S, ten Cate JM, Angmar-Månsson B, de Josselin de Jong E, Sundström G, Exterkate RA, et al. Quantification of formation and remineralization of artificial enamel lesions with a new portable fluorescence device. Adv Dent Res. 1997 Nov;11(4):502–6.

47. Hall AF, DeSchepper E, Ando M, Stookey GK. In vitro studies of laser fluorescence for detection and quantification of mineral loss from dental caries. Adv Dent Res. 1997 Nov;11(4):507–14.

48. Ando M, Hall AF, Eckert GJ, Schemehorn BR, Analoui M, Stookey GK. Relative ability of laser fluorescence techniques to quantitate early mineral loss in vitro. Caries Res. 1997;31(2):125–31.

49. Lagerweij M, van der Veen M, Ando M, Lukantsova L, Stookey G. The validity and repeatability of three light-induced fluorescence systems: An in vitro study. Caries Res. 1999;33(3):220–6.

50. Detection of Occlusal Caries by Laser Fluorescence: Basic and Clinical Investigations - ScienceDirect [Internet]. [cited 2024 Jan 29].

51. König K, Flemming G, Hibst R. Laser-induced autofluorescence spectroscopy of dental caries. Cell Mol Biol (Noisy-le-grand). 1998 Dec;44(8):1293–300.

52. Performance and reproducibility of a laser fluorescence system for detection of occlusal caries in vitro - PubMed [Internet]. [cited 2024 Jan 29].

53. Pitts NB. Diagnostic tools and measurements--impact on appropriate care. Community Dent Oral Epidemiol. 1997 Feb;25(1):24–35.

54. Davies G, Worthington H, Clarkson J, Thomas P, Davies R. The use of fibre-optic transillumination in general dental practice. British dental journal. 2001 Sep 1;191:145–7.

55. Peers A, Hill FJ, Mitropoulos CM, Holloway PJ. Validity and reproducibility of clinical examination, fibre-optic transillumination, and bite-wing radiology for the diagnosis of small approximal carious lesions: an in vitro study. Caries Res. 1993;27(4):307–11.

56. Longbottom C, Huysmans MC, Pitts NB, Los P, Bruce PG. Detection of dental decay and its extent using a.c. impedance spectroscopy. Nat Med. 1996 Feb;2(2):235–7.

57. Verdonschot EH, Angmar-Månsson B, ten Bosch JJ, Deery CH, Huysmans MC, Pitts NB, et al. Developments in caries diagnosis and their relationship to treatment decisions and quality of care. ORCA Saturday Afternoon Symposium 1997. Caries Res. 1999;33(1):32–40.

58. Application of magnetic resonance microimaging to the study of dental caries - PubMed [Internet]. [cited 2024 Jan 29].

59. Fusayama T. Two layers of carious dentin; diagnosis and treatment. Oper Dent. 1979;4(2):63–70.

60. Kuboki Y, Liu CF, Fusayama T. Mechanism of differential staining in carious dentin. J Dent Res. 1983 Jun;62(6):713–4.

61. Fusayama T. Clinical guide for removing caries using a caries-detecting solution. Quintessence Int. 1988 Jun;19(6):397–401.

62. Anderson MH, Charbeneau GT. A comparison of digital and optical criteria for detecting carious dentin. J Prosthet Dent. 1985 May;53(5):643–6.

63. Kidd EA, Joyston-Bechal S, Smith MM, Allan R, Howe L, Smith SR. The use of a caries detector dye in cavity preparation. Br Dent J. 1989 Aug 19;167(4):132–4.

64. Use of dyes in cariology - PubMed [Internet]. [cited 2024 Jan 29].

65. The Efficiency of Operating Microscope Compared with Unaided Visual Examination, Conventional and Digital Intraoral Radiography for Proximal Caries Detection [Internet]. [cited 2024 Jan 29].

66. Jc A. Pulp effects of neodymium laser. A preliminary report. Oral surgery, oral medicine, and oral pathology [Internet]. 1977 Aug [cited 2024 Jan 29];44(2).

67. Smales RJ, Yip HK. The atraumatic restorative treatment (ART) approach for primary teeth: review of literature. Pediatr Dent. 2000;22(4):294–8.

68. Li J, Helmerhorst EJ, Leone CW, Troxler RF, Yaskell T, Haffajee AD, et al. Identification of early microbial colonizers in human dental biofilm. J Appl Microbiol. 2004;97(6):1311–8.

69. Larsen MJ. Chemical events during tooth dissolution. J Dent Res. 1990 Feb;69 Spec No:575–80; discussion 634-636.

70. Gorelick L, Geiger AM, Gwinnett AJ. Incidence of white spot formation after bonding and banding. American Journal of Orthodontics. 1982 Feb 1;81(2):93–8.

71. The caries balance: the basis for caries management by risk assessment - PubMed [Internet]. [cited 2024 Mar 1].

72. Simonsen RJ. Pit and fissure sealant: review of the literature. Pediatric Dentistry. 2002;

73. Fundamentals of Pediatric Dentistry [3 ed.] 0867152621, 9780867152623 [Internet]. dokumen.pub. [cited 2024 Mar 1].

74. Textbook of Pedodontics - Google Books [Internet]. [cited 2024 Mar 1].

75. Williams B, Laxton L, Holt RD, Winter GB. Fissure sealants: a 4-year clinical trial comparing an experimental glass polyalkenoate cement with a bis glycidyl methacrylate resin used as fissure sealants. Br Dent J. 1996 Feb 10;180(3):104–8.

76. Sathyaprasad DS. MINI IMPLANTS IN PEDIATRIC DENTISTRY- A REVIEW. International Journal of Current Research. 2020;12.

77. Savitha s, havaldar k. Mini implants in pediatric dentistry -a review. 2022 feb 27

78. Inlays & Onlays - An Alternative to Traditional Fillings and Crowns [Internet]. [cited 2024 Mar 2].

79. Mahadevan G, Parikh D. Chemomechanical caries removal (CMCR) agents: Review and clinical application in primary teeth. J Dent Oral Hyg. 2010 Nov 30;3.

80. Boob AR, Manjula M, Reddy ER, Srilaxmi N, Rani T. Evaluation of the Efficiency and Effectiveness of Three Minimally Invasive Methods of Caries Removal: An in vitro Study. Int J Clin Pediatr Dent. 2014;7(1):11–8.

81. Burke FM, Lynch E. Chemomechanical caries removal. J Ir Dent Assoc. 1995;41(1):10–4.

82. Beeley JA, Yip HK, Stevenson AG. Chemochemical caries removal: a review of the techniques and latest developments. Br Dent J. 2000 Apr 22;188(8):427–30.

83. Yip HK, Smales RJ. Glass ionomer cements used as fissure sealants with the atraumatic restorative treatment (ART) approach: review of literature. Int Dent J. 2002 Apr;52(2):67–70.

84. Paurazas SB, Geist JR, Pink FE, Hoen MM, Steiman HR. Comparison of diagnostic accuracy of digital imaging by using CCD and CMOS-APS sensors with E-speed film in the detection of periapical bony lesions. Oral Surg Oral Med Oral Pathol Oral Radiol Endod. 2000 Mar;89(3):356–62.

85. Digital radiography and caries diagnosis - PubMed [Internet]. [cited 2024 Mar 2].

86. Møystad A, Svanaes DB, Risnes S, Larheim TA, Gröndahl HG. Detection of approximal caries with a storage phosphor system. A comparison of enhanced digital images with dental X-ray film. Dentomaxillofac Radiol. 1996 Sep;25(4):202–6.

87. Cederberg RA, Tidwell E, Frederiksen NL, Benson BW. Endodontic working length assessment. Comparison of storage phosphor digital imaging and radiographic film. Oral Surg Oral Med Oral Pathol Oral Radiol Endod. 1998 Mar;85(3):325–8.

88. Digital imaging for dental caries - ScienceDirect [Internet]. [cited 2024 Mar 2].

89. Ericson D, Kidd E, McComb D, Mjör I, Noack MJ. Minimally Invasive Dentistry--concepts and techniques in cariology. Oral Health Prev Dent. 2003;1(1):59–72.

90. Olivi G, Genovese MD, Caprioglio C. Evidence-based dentistry on laser paediatric dentistry: review and outlook. Eur J Paediatr Dent. 2009 Mar;10(1):29–40.

91. Indications and limitations of Er:YAG laser applications in dentistry - PubMed [Internet]. [cited 2024 Mar 2].

92. Tassery H, Koubi S. Minimally Invasive Dentistry Using Sonic and Ultra-sonic Devices in Ultraconservative Class 2 Restorations. The Journal of Contemporary Dental Practice. 2008 Feb;9(2):155–65.

93. Minimally Invasive Dentistry Using Sonic and Ultra-sonic Devices in Ultraconservative Class 2 Restorations | Request PDF. ResearchGate [Internet]. [cited 2023 Nov 8];

94. Rickard GD, Richardson RJ, Johnson TM, McColl DC, Hooper L. Ozone therapy for the treatment of dental caries. Cochrane Database of Systematic Reviews [Internet]. 2004 [cited 2023 Nov 8];(3).

95. Ozone therapy in dentistry: A strategic review.

96. Kornman K, Polverini P. Clinical application of genetics to guide prevention and treatment of oral diseases. Clin Genet. 2014 Jan;86(1):44–9.

97. Genetically modified Streptococcus mutans for the prevention of dental caries.

98. The Role of Matrix Metalloproteinases (MMPs) in Human Caries - C. Chaussain-Miller, F. Fioretti, M. Goldberg, S. Menashi, 2006 [Internet].

99. New Technological Approaches for Dental Caries Treatment: From Liquid Crystalline Systems to Nanocarriers.

100. Alyahya Y. A narrative review of minimally invasive techniques in restorative dentistry. The Saudi Dental Journal. 2024 Feb 1;36(2):228–33.

FSC
www.fsc.org
MIX
Papier | Fördert
gute Waldnutzung
FSC® C083411

Kolibri 360 GmbH
Ferdinand-Jühlke-Straße 7
99095 Erfurt, Deutschland
produktsicherheit@kolibri360.de

Druck:
CPI Druckdienstleistungen GmbH
im Auftrag der
Kolibri 360 GmbH
Ferdinand-Jühlke-Str. 7
99095 Erfurt